VIROLOGY RESEARCH PROGRESS

SWINE FLU

SIGNS/SYMPTOMS, PREVENTIVE METHODS AND TREATMENT OPTIONS

VIROLOGY RESEARCH PROGRESS

Additional books in this series can be found on Nova's website
under the Series tab.

Additional E-books in this series can be found on Nova's website
under the E-book tab.

PUBLIC HEALTH IN THE 21ST CENTURY

Additional books in this series can be found on Nova's website
under the Series tab.

Additional E-books in this series can be found on Nova's website
under the E-book tab.

VIROLOGY RESEARCH PROGRESS

SWINE FLU

SIGNS/SYMPTOMS, PREVENTIVE METHODS AND TREATMENT OPTIONS

JULIA C. MARIE
AND
THOMAS B. JOHNSON
EDITORS

NOVINKA

New York

LIBRARY OF CONGRESS CATALOGING-IN-PUBLICATION DATA

ISBN: 978-1-62618-363-6

Library of Congress Control Number: 2013933837

Published by Nova Science Publishers, Inc. † New York

CONTENTS

PREFACE

Swine-origin influenza A (H1N1), better known as swine flu, was declared by the World Health Organization as a global pandemic in June 2009. The highly contagious influenza A H1N1 virus can cause either a mild influenza-like infection that is similar to seasonal influenza, or less frequently, a rapidly progressing community-acquired pneumonic illness that can cause acute respiratory failure and even death. This book addresses the signs/symptoms, epidemiology, preventive methods and treatment options for swine flu.

Chapter 1 – Influenza is an acute respiratory viral infectious illness that is universally distributed and has a high capacity to spread and disseminate, impacting the morbidity and mortality of specific population groups. It is transmitted by air, contaminated fomites or close contact. The swine flu pandemic that occurred in 2009 was a global outbreak that affected more than 20 countries. According to published studies, most infected individuals showed mild symptoms, with clinical recovery within a few days. More than 50% of those infected were young patients below 50 years, 50% had no underlying disease, 30% were obese and 10% were pregnant women. The pathogenesis, in general, is similar to the normal flu (cough, runny nose, high fever, malaise, headache, eye and pharyngeal pain, arthralgia, myalgia, asthenia and, in some cases, diarrhea and nausea), progressing to spontaneous healing. However, there is a wide clinical spectrum, from an asymptomatic presentation to severe pneumonia or death. It occasionally shows rapid evolution (in approximately 5 days) to pneumonia and acute respiratory distress, fulminating in half the cases. Studies have shown that the swine flu infection can cause serious pulmonary complications in young people without comorbidities, especially children, who show the highest rates of hospitalization. Preventing the spread of influenza A H1N1 can be accomplished similar to the common flu and is based on hand hygiene and avoiding local clustering. The currently available treatment includes two classes of drugs: inhibitors of the M2 ion channel (amantadine and rimantadine) and neuraminidase (NA) inhibitors (zanamivir and oseltamivir). An initial analysis showed that the new swine flu strain of influenza A (H1N1) was sensitive to NA inhibitors but resistant to amantadine and rimantadine. A NA inhibitor that is under investigation is peramivir. These drugs can be administered either in a preventive manner to individuals who come into contact with a high-risk population or to treat people infected with influenza A H1N1. The purpose of this chapter is to review published information about swine flu, including its signs and symptoms, prevention and available treatment options.

Chapter 2 – Influenza is one of the most common infections worldwide. It often causes a life-threatening illness in humans. The pandemic of 2009 is still fresh in our memory.

While a large amount of information concerning the natural history and clinical management of 2009 H1N1 virus infection has been obtained in a remarkably short period, there are several medical problems still remaining.

They are; analyzing risk factors among patients with swine flu for severe illness, the effectiveness of vaccination, the management for swine flu and its complications, the emergence of oseltamivir-resistant influenza virus and therapeutic options such as extracorporeal membrane oxygenation (ECMO) and traditional herbal medicine.

This chapter describes the epidemiology, clinical manifestations, risk factors, preventive methods, treatment options and new topics on swine flu.

Chapter 3 – Influenza - A virus of swine origin, H1N1, is a highly contagious virus that has been rapidly transmitted and spread among humans in many countries causing a global pandemic. Clinical manifestations of disease range from asymptomatic infection to mild upper respiratory illness, or severe pneumonia to acute respiratory distress syndrome (ARDS) with progression to multi-organ failure, and an adverse outcome. Populations at increased risk for morbidity and mortality include the very young and elderly, the pregnant, individuals with comorbid chronic cardiopulmonary conditions, and the immunocompromized. In early stages or in mild cases of infection, chest radiographs can appear normal. With progression of lung infection, typical radiographic and CT findings of the H1N1 viral infection include bilateral, multifocal areas of consolidation associated with ground-glass opacities, in the absence of pleural effusion or lymphadenopathy. Experience from many clinical cases has shown that extensive involvement of both lungs is invariably associated with an adverse prognosis. Recognition of the imaging findings of lung infection (albeit nonspecific for H1N1 viral pneumonia) when associated with clinical and laboratory results may have significance, in the prediction of clinical outcome.

Chapter 4 – During the outburst of Influenza A H1N1 in China in 2009, our hospital admitted 232 confirmed cases of Influenza A H1N1, including 67 cases of severely ill patients. All of the 67 severe Influenza A H1N1 cases combined with pneumonia, with 6 cases of unilateral pneumonia and 61 cases of double pneumonia. This section enumerated five typical severely ill cases of Influenza A H1N1, including the combination of respiratory failure and fungal infections, hemophagocytic syndrome, invasive pulmonary aspergillosis, pericardial effusion, and pregnancy. All of the 67 cases of severe Influenza A H1N1 have been successfully cured, except one case of pregnant woman. Herein, the curing methods for the 5 typical severe cases were discussed, with the summarized treatment experiences. The early treatment was with the great importance for the curing of severely ill patients of Influenza A H1N1, and efficient monitoring and treatment could prevent the mild Influenza A H1N1 developing to severe conditions. Ventilator supporting and glucocorticoids treatment could be used for curing of Influenza A H1N1infection at specific indicators.

Chapter 5 – During summer and autumn of 2009, Norway, like several other European countries, experienced an unexpected delay in the emergence and spread of the new pandemic influenza A (H1N1)pdm09. It is considered whether interference of other respiratory viruses, in particular rhinoviruses, may have hampered the development of the pandemic, and if interference phenomena are common in the development of outbreaks with epidemic viruses. If so, cytokines, in particular interferon, are the most probable executor of this effect. The virus interference theory may form a reasonable explanation why pandemic influenza, in contrast to seasonal influenza, tends to occur in waves.

In: Swine Flu
Editors: J. C. Marie and T. B. Johnson
ISBN: 978-1-62618-363-6

Chapter 1

TREATMENT OPTIONS FOR SWINE FLU

Luana Lenzi, Astrid Wiens and Roberto Pontarolo*
Departamento de Farmácia, Universidade Federal do Paraná,
Jardim Botânico, Curitiba, PR, Brasil

ABSTRACT

Influenza is an acute respiratory viral infectious illness that is universally distributed and has a high capacity to spread and disseminate, impacting the morbidity and mortality of specific population groups. It is transmitted by air, contaminated fomites or close contact. The swine flu pandemic that occurred in 2009 was a global outbreak that affected more than 20 countries. According to published studies, most infected individuals showed mild symptoms, with clinical recovery within a few days. More than 50% of those infected were young patients below 50 years, 50% had no underlying disease, 30% were obese and 10% were pregnant women. The pathogenesis, in general, is similar to the normal flu (cough, runny nose, high fever, malaise, headache, eye and pharyngeal pain, arthralgia, myalgia, asthenia and, in some cases, diarrhea and nausea), progressing to spontaneous healing. However, there is a wide clinical spectrum, from an asymptomatic presentation to severe pneumonia or death. It occasionally shows rapid evolution (in approximately 5 days) to pneumonia and acute respiratory distress, fulminating in half the cases. Studies have shown that the swine flu infection can cause serious pulmonary complications in young people

* E-mail: pontarolo@ufpr.br.

without comorbidities, especially children, who show the highest rates of hospitalization. Preventing the spread of influenza A H1N1 can be accomplished similar to the common flu and is based on hand hygiene and avoiding local clustering. The currently available treatment includes two classes of drugs: inhibitors of the M2 ion channel (amantadine and rimantadine) and neuraminidase (NA) inhibitors (zanamivir and oseltamivir). An initial analysis showed that the new swine flu strain of influenza A (H1N1) was sensitive to NA inhibitors but resistant to amantadine and rimantadine. A NA inhibitor that is under investigation is peramivir. These drugs can be administered either in a preventive manner to individuals who come into contact with a high-risk population or to treat people infected with influenza A H1N1. The purpose of this chapter is to review published information about swine flu, including its signs and symptoms, prevention and available treatment options.

INTRODUCTION

Influenza is an acute respiratory viral infectious illness that is universally distributed and has a high capacity to spread and disseminate, impacting the morbidity and mortality of specific population groups. It is transmitted by air, contaminated fomites or close contact. The swine flu pandemic that occurred in 2009 rapidly spread throughout the world and was a global outbreak that affected more than 200 countries. In June 2009, the World Health Organization (WHO) raised the alert level to phase 6. According to published studies, most of those infected showed mild symptoms, with clinical recovery in a few days. Over 50% of those infected were young patients below 50 years, 50% had underlying disease, 30% were obese and 10% were pregnant women. The pathogenesis, in general, is similar to the normal flu (cough, runny nose, high fever, malaise, headache, eye and pharyngeal pain, arthralgia, myalgia, asthenia and, in some cases, diarrhea and nausea), progressing to spontaneous healing. However, there is a wide clinical spectrum, from an asymptomatic presentation to severe pneumonia or death. Occasionally, it shows rapid evolution (in approximately 5 days) to pneumonia and acute respiratory distress, fulminating in half the cases. Studies have shown that the swine flu infection can cause serious pulmonary complications in young people without comorbidities, especially in children, who have the highest rates of hospitalization. Preventing the spread of influenza A H1N1 can be accomplished similar to the common flu and is based on hand hygiene and avoiding local clustering. The currently available treatment includes two classes of drugs: inhibitors of the M2 ion channel (amantadine and rimantadine) and NA inhibitors (zanamivir and oseltamivir). An initial analysis showed that the new swine flu strain of influenza A (H1N1) was sensitive to NA inhibitors but resistant to amantadine and rimantadine. A NA inhibitor that is under investigation is peramivir. These drugs can be administered either in a preventive manner to individuals who came into contact with a high-risk population or to treat people infected with influenza A H1N1. The purpose of this chapter is to review published information about swine flu, including its signs and symptoms, prevention and available treatment options.

Swine Flu

Of the various respiratory diseases, influenza is a major cause of mortality and morbidity among patients, particularly the very young, the elderly and persons of any age who have medical conditions that place them at increased risk for complications from influenza [1-3]. In the postpandemic period, 2009 H1N1 virus strains are now considered to be the predominant seasonal influenza A (H1N1) virus strains [4].

In most cases, the clinical signs are mild and similar to those observed with seasonal influenza infections, typically including fever, cough and sore throat [5]. However, some patients may progress to severe, progressive or complicated illness. Clinical and observational data show that early antiviral treatment can shorten the duration of fever and illness symptoms, reduce the risk of complications from influenza and shorten the duration of hospitalization.

Antiviral Treatment

Most cases of influenza are self-limited, and prevention through annual influenza vaccination may be an effective strategy. Antiviral medications are effective for the prevention of influenza, and when used for early treatment, they can reduce the duration and severity of illness and reduce the risk for severe illness or death related to influenza [4, 6-8].

Antiviral treatment options include the NA inhibitors (oseltamivir, zanamivir, laninamivir, and peramivir) and M2 ion channel blockers (amantadine or rimantadine). A review of antivirals, including their indications, adverse reactions and resistance, is presented in the following sections.

Adamantanes

Amantadine and rimantadine are related antiviral drugs in a class of medications known as adamantanes. These medications are active against influenza A viruses but not influenza B viruses and are associated with several toxic effects and the rapid emergence of drug-resistant variants. Adamantanes interfere with viral uncoating inside the cell.

The pandemic influenza A (H1N1) 2009 virus was initially found to be susceptible to NA inhibitors but resistant to adamantanes [9].

In recent years, widespread adamantane resistance among influenza A (H3N2) virus strains has made this class of medications less useful clinically. The emergence of pathogenic, transmissible, and amantadine-resistant H1N1 and H3N2 seasonal influenza variants, amantadine resistance in the pandemic H1N1 2009 influenza viruses, and a significant increase in amantadine resistance among some highly pathogenic H5N1 viruses have limited the usefulness of M2 ion channel blockers [10-12]. Therefore, amantadine and rimantadine are not recommended for the antiviral treatment or chemoprophylaxis of currently circulating influenza A virus strains.

Neuraminidase Inhibitors

Because of the increase in resistance to amantadine and rimantadine and the lack of an effective vaccine, NA inhibitors have become a widespread public health intervention. NA inhibitors are considered an important strategy to limit the impact of an influenza pandemic by reducing morbidity and mortality and, collectively, by slowing the spread of the virus to allow time for vaccine production, the cornerstone of influenza control [13-15].

These medications are active against both influenza A and B viruses. NA inhibitors interfere with the release of progeny influenza virus from infected host cells, which prevents the infection of new host cells and thereby halts the spread of infection in the respiratory tract. In contrast to adamantanes, NA inhibitors are associated with little toxicity and are far less likely to lead to the development of drug-resistant influenza [16].

The use of NA inhibitors has increased dramatically with the spread of the influenza A/H1N1 pandemic that began in April 2009, a novel and potentially serious infection [17]. Because influenza virus replication in the respiratory tract reaches its peak between 24 and 72 hours after the onset of the illness, drugs, such as NA inhibitors, that act at the stage of viral replication must be administered as early as possible [16].

As a class, NA inhibitors are effective against all NA subtypes and, therefore, against all strains of influenza, a key point in epidemic and pandemic preparedness and an important advantage over adamantanes, which are only effective against sensitive strains of influenza A. These drugs, if used properly, have great potential for diminishing the effects of influenza infection [16].

The ability of transition-state analogues of sialic acid to inhibit influenza NA was first recognized in the 1970s [18-20], but the design of highly effective inhibitors became feasible when an analysis of the three-dimensional structure of influenza NA 6 showed the location and structure of the catalytic site. Potent inhibitors, such as zanamivir, closely mimic the natural substrate, fitting into the active site pocket and engaging the protein in the most energetically favorable interaction [21-23].

Oseltamivir

Oseltamivir (Tamiflu; F. Hoffmann-La Roche Ltd) is FDA approved for the treatment and chemoprophylaxis of adults and children aged >1 year of age with uncomplicated acute illness caused by influenza A or B virus [24]. Emergency authorization has recently been granted in several countries for use in infants <1 year old with pandemic (H1N1) 2009. According to guidance from the WHO, the CDC and the European Centre for Disease Prevention and Control (ECDC) [5, 25-27], oseltamivir treatment should be used in patients with severe disease caused by the pandemic virus and in recognized groups of high-risk patients (children aged < 5 years, pregnant women, adults over 65 years, immunosuppressed patients and those with concomitant diseases).

Oseltamivir was developed through modifications to the sialic acid analogue framework (including the addition of a lipophilic side chain), which allow the drug to be used orally. It is prescribed twice per day in divided dosages for 5 days (4 mg/kg/day, maximum of 150 mg/day) [28].

Oseltamivir is available for oral administration in 30 mg, 45 mg, and 75 mg capsules and liquid suspension, both of which have good oral bioavailability. It is readily absorbed from the gastrointestinal tract, converted by hepatic esterases to oseltamivir carboxylate, the active form of the compound, and widely distributed in the body. The half-life is 6 to 10 hours. The drug is excreted primarily through the kidneys; thus, dosing must be modified in patients with renal insufficiency. Oseltamivir achieves high plasma levels and can act outside the respiratory tract [4,16].

Serum concentrations of oseltamivir carboxylate increase with declining renal function [24]. For patients with creatinine clearance of 10–30 mL per minute, a reduction of the treatment dosage of oseltamivir to 75 mg once daily and the chemoprophylactic dosage to 75 mg every other day is recommended [24, 29].

NA inhibitors are thought to be efficacious compared to placebo in outpatients with uncomplicated seasonal influenza [15,17,30], both clinically in terms of a reduction in the duration of symptoms and in terms of a reduction in viral shedding. One large study evaluated the efficacy of oseltamivir treatment in 629 healthy, nonimmunized adults 18 to 65 years of age who presented with a febrile respiratory illness of no more than 36 hours duration and one respiratory and one constitutional symptom. Oseltamivir treatment reduced the median duration of illness by more than 30 percent (from 4.3 days to 3 days) and the severity of illness by approximately 40 percent. There was a reduction in fever and a resolution of symptoms as soon as 24 hours after the initiation of treatment. Furthermore, treated patients had a lower frequency of secondary complications than untreated patients [31].

The early initiation of treatment (within 48 hours of symptoms) appears to be the most important determinant of treatment efficacy, although initiation after 48 hours is considered beneficial. Treatment that began within the first 12 hours after the onset of fever shortened the illness by more than 3 days compared with treatment that was started at 48 hours. The initiation of treatment at intermediate times shortened the illness proportionately. The duration of fever, the severity of symptoms, and the time to return to normal activity also correlated with the time of antiviral intervention, leading to the clear conclusion that treatment initiated at 36 to 48 hours after the onset of symptoms does not show the excellent outcomes obtained with earlier treatment [25-27, 32].

The early administration of the drug within 12 hours after the onset of symptoms appreciably increased the effectiveness of oseltamivir therapy for both influenza A and B, suggesting that the prompt identification of illness and the initiation of treatment as early as possible should be the goal for the proper use of NA inhibitors [16].

Oseltamivir has few adverse effects when administered for either treatment or prophylaxis. The most frequent side effects are transient nausea, vomiting, and abdominal pain, which occur in approximately 5 to 10 percent of patients. Most adverse events occur only once, close to the initiation of therapy, and resolve spontaneously within one to two days. The safety profile among elderly persons is similar to that in persons younger than 65 years. The consumption of food does not interfere with the absorption of oseltamivir and may reduce nausea and vomiting [33,34].

The development of resistance is a major obstacle to the usefulness of both classes of anti-influenza agents, which could provide a growth advantage to variants carrying drug-resistance mutations, more likely under drug-selective pressure. The published frequency of viruses that were isolated after treatment and resistant to the drug is higher. Approximately 0.4 percent of treated adults harbored viruses with resistant NAs. The NA inhibitor resistance-associated mutations in influenza viruses are drug specific and NA subtype specific [16, 35,36].

The NA inhibitor-resistant variants differ in fitness and transmissibility, which are influenced by the location of NA mutation(s) [37,38], indicating that transmissible NA inhibitor-resistant variants may emerge. Therefore, continuous monitoring is necessary [36]. Until 2007, influenza viruses resistant to the NA inhibitor oseltamivir were isolated at a low level. However, during the 2007-2008 influenza season, oseltamivir-resistant variants with the H275Y NA amino acid substitution (N1 numbering) became widespread, first in the Northern Hemisphere [39,40] and then in the Southern Hemisphere [41]. Sporadic oseltamivir-resistant 2009 H1N1 virus infections have been identified, including in rare episodes of limited transmission [42-46], but the public health impact has been limited to date. However, additional sporadic cases of oseltamivir-resistant 2009 H1N1 virus infection can be expected, and ongoing surveillance for oseltamivir resistance among influenza viruses is essential for public health because oseltamivir is the treatment agent favored by clinicians and is the most widely used antiviral medication [4].

Zanamivir

Zanamivir (Relenza; GlaxoSmithKline) is approved by the U.S. FDA for use against type A and type B influenza infections in adults with uncomplicated acute illness and children aged ≥7 years and for the chemoprophylaxis of influenza among adults and children aged ≥5 years. The treatment and chemoprophylaxis dosing and frequency are the same for children and adults, but zanamivir is not recommended for persons with underlying airways disease (e.g., asthma or chronic obstructive pulmonary diseases) [47].

Zanamivir is administered by oral inhalation with a dry powder inhaler device in 5 mg blister doses per inhalation, which delivers the drug directly to the respiratory tract. The recommended dosage of zanamivir for influenza treatment is inhalations (5 mg blister per inhalation for a total dose of 10 mg) twice daily (approximately 12 hours apart) for 5 days. The chemoprophylactic dosage of zanamivir is 10 mg (2 inhalations) once a day. No reduction in the dosage of zanamivir is recommended on the basis of age alone [47].

Zanamivir is highly concentrated in the respiratory tract; 10 to 20 percent of the active compound reaches the lungs, and the rest is deposited in the oropharynx. The bioavailability of the drug is 10-20% by inhalation compared with 2% by oral administration, a feature that is potentially advantageous in situations in which a systemic drug is undesirable. Approximately 90% of the absorbed dose is excreted unchanged in the urine. The concentration of the drug in the respiratory tract has been estimated to be more than 1000 times as high as the 50 percent inhibitory concentration (IC50) for NA; in addition, the inhibitory effect starts within 10 seconds — two favorable features in terms of reducing the likelihood of the emergence of drug-resistant variant viruses [16].

The poor oral bioavailability of zanamivir (~2%) is well documented [48] and provides an impetus for the development of alternate administration routes for the drug. Investigational preparations of zanamivir that can be administered parenterally have been reported to reduce the likelihood of infection in a challenge model of experimental infection with influenza A virus [4, 49]. In healthy volunteers receiving 600 mg zanamivir or placebo intravenously twice daily for 5 days prior to a virus challenge, zanamivir was found to be highly protective against experimental infection (14% vs. 100%, respectively, were infected), reduce viral shedding (0% vs. 100%, respectively, had viral shedding), and prevent illness [50]. Intravenous zanamivir has been used with success in clinical settings [51,52] and is the recommended antiviral treatment for severely ill patients with highly suspected or confirmed oseltamivir-resistant 2009 H1N1 virus infection [51,53,54]. Intravenous zanamivir was active in a primate model of influenza A (H5N1) virus infection, and the Southeast Asia Influenza Clinical Research Network is developing a protocol to study it in patients with avian influenza A (H5N1) illness [55,56].

For patients who are intubated, using the zanamivir disc inhaler is not possible. Suboptimal delivery to sites of infection in patients with pneumonic or extrapulmonary disease is also of concern for patients with severe respiratory illness [49]. The limited experimental use of an unlicensed nebulized formulation of zanamivir has been well tolerated [57], but use of the nebulized preparation of the licensed powder formulation contained in the disc inhaler is not recommended because it has been demonstrated to clog ventilator tubing [58]. A 4-week study in community-dwelling persons at higher risk for influenza complications (median age: 60 years) demonstrated that zanamivir showed 83% effectiveness in preventing symptomatic laboratory-confirmed influenza [59].

Zanamivir and oseltamivir are similar in their mode of action, but the drugs have different structural and biochemical properties, which influences their route of administration. NAIs target the active site of the NA protein, inhibiting its sialidase activity, which is essential for virus release [60]. The first antivirals directed against NA were rationally designed on the basis of the X-ray crystal structure of N2-type NAs (i.e., N2 and N9). NA is a tetramer, and each monomer has a sialic acid-binding pocket lined by amino acids that are conserved in all influenza A and B virus strains. A sialic acid derivative in which the 4-hydroxyl group of sialic acid is replaced with a guanidinyl group binds to this pocket tighter than sialic acid itself. The resulting compound, zanamivir, effectively inhibits the NA of influenza A and B viruses and is orders of magnitude less active against non-influenza NAs [61].

In general, zanamivir is well tolerated; studies to date suggest that adverse effects, primarily minor, transient upper respiratory and gastrointestinal symptoms, develop in equal numbers of patients in drug and placebo groups. However, post-licensure reports indicate that zanamivir may cause cough, bronchospasm, and a reversible decrease in pulmonary function in some patients [16,62]. The most common adverse events reported in more than 1.5% of all patients treated with zanamivir are sinusitis and dizziness. In addition, there have been reports of fatal respiratory complications, such as bronchospasm, following the inhalation of zanamivir. Neuropsychiatric events have also been reported, particularly in the pediatric age group [60].

Limited data are available regarding the safety and efficacy of zanamivir in patients with impaired renal function. Among patients with renal failure who were administered a single intravenous dose of zanamivir, decreases in renal clearance, increases in the half-life, and increased systemic exposure to zanamivir were reported [24]. However, a limited number of healthy volunteers who were administered high doses of intravenous zanamivir tolerated systemic levels of zanamivir that were substantially higher than those resulting from the administration of zanamivir by oral inhalation at the recommended dose [50, 63]. On the basis of these considerations, the manufacturer recommends no dose adjustment for inhaled zanamivir for a 5-day course of treatment for patients with mild-to-moderate or severe impairment in renal function [47]. In contrast, a well-controlled trial demonstrated that the recommended dosages of zanamivir did not adversely affect pulmonary function in patients with respiratory disorders [64]. If patients with pulmonary dysfunction do receive zanamivir, it is recommended that they have a fast-acting bronchodilator available and discontinue zanamivir if respiratory difficulty develops [16].

Oseltamivir is easier to administer and has therefore been more widely used than zanamivir. For this reason, most of the literature on antiviral resistance associated with NAIs has only investigated antiviral resistance associated with oseltamivir. The isolation of influenza A viruses with reduced susceptibility to zanamivir has rarely been reported. To date, influenza A and B, including all types of influenza A H1N1 virus, remain susceptible to zanamivir. Clinical isolates with reduced susceptibility to zanamivir have occasionally been obtained from immunocompromised children on prolonged therapy. However, due to the higher resistance rates associated with oseltamivir, especially for influenza A H1N1 strains between 2007-09, zanamivir has been increasingly utilized for the treatment and prevention of influenza. It has been proposed that zanamivir should be reserved for the treatment of cases of 2009 H1N1 that are resistant to oseltamivir. Therefore, there is a need to investigate the development of influenza resistance to zanamivir during this time [65-69].

All these resistant viruses had the same amino acid substitution, His274Tyr, in their NA protein, which had no apparent effect on the fitness of the virus. H5N1 and H1N1 viruses with the His274Tyr mutant NA remained susceptible to zanamivir, demonstrating that even if such mutant viruses became predominant, at least one NA inhibitor would still be potent [61].

Peramivir

Peramivir is a potent investigational NA inhibitor that selectively inhibits the NA of human type A and type B influenza viruses. It may also have potent NA inhibitory activity against highly pathogenic influenza viruses. Additionally, it can inhibit NA activity for long periods [70,71]. Peramivir consists of a cyclopentane backbone with a positively charged guanidinyl group and lipophilic side chains [72].

Peramivir is generally well tolerated and shows improvement of symptoms at 24 hours after administration. The indicated doses of administration are between 300 and 600 mg intravenously in a single dose. Multiple doses of peramivir are effective for high-risk patients for complications. The drug was made available when the U.S. Food and Drug Administration authorized peramivir exclusively for severe pandemic H1N1, and this authorized regimen was 600 mg/day for 5 to 10 days [70,71,73]. During this period, the drug was administered to 20 adults and 11 children. It was well tolerated and associated with recovery in most of the included patients [74].

In a randomized controlled trial in pediatric patients, peramivir 10 mg/kg was administered to children infected with pH1N1 virus. High therapeutic efficacy was observed, and the pediatric patients recuperated twice as rapidly, when compared with untreated patients. The most frequently reported adverse event was a decrease in neutrophil count, which was severe in 10 patients [73].

Peramivir is only available in the U. S. through participation in an ongoing phase 3 trial. It is already approved in Japan and Korea for the treatment of influenza. Given the serious health threat of influenza and limitations in vaccine delivery, peramivir is a promising addition to the currently limited treatment options for the treatment of severe influenza infection [72].

Laninamivir

Laninamivir octanoate is a promising influenza NA inhibitor with high potency. It is a prodrug of laninamivir, which inhibit the NA activities of various influenza A and B viruses and the pandemic 2009 H1N1 virus. This NA inhibitor has a long duration of action, and it exerts beneficial effects by remaining in the target organs (trachea and lungs) for a long time [75,76].

In a comparative study between laninamivir and oseltamivir, the median time to influenza A (H1N1) alleviation was similar in both groups. Complications and rates of exacerbation were also similar in both groups. The authors concluded that a single inhalation of laninamivir octanoate can be used safely for the treatment of influenza [75].

Laninamivir octanoate was compared with zanamivir in pediatric patients, with similar results of efficiency and safety in both groups. However, the advantage of using laninamivir is that it required only a single inhalation [77].

Laninamivir has been approved in Japan [78], but there are no records of the approval of this drug by the FDA.

Combination of Antiviral Agents

It was hypothesized that the widespread use of a single antiviral might result in the emergence of resistant strains whose subsequent spread could dramatically reduce the effectiveness of antiviral therapy. An attractive approach for countering drug resistance is combination chemotherapy with two or more drugs that target different viral proteins or host factors and for which the mechanisms of resistance differ.

The combination of two antiviral agents, if well tolerated and producing at least additive antiviral activity, theoretically offers several advantages, including reducing the disease severity, viral shedding, and viral excretion period, thereby decreasing the attack rate and risk of selection of resistant viruses, especially in individuals with prolonged viral shedding, such as immunocompromised patients.

Another theoretical advantage of combining two drugs would be to ensure the optimal treatment of all circulating influenza virus types, subtypes, or variants, as the susceptibility of influenza viruses has been shown to vary, and seasonal H1N1 viruses that were naturally resistant to oseltamivir but remained susceptible to zanamivir emerged in 2008. Moreover, combination therapy may not only potentiate antiviral activity but also enhance clinical outcomes by allowing reductions of the doses of individual drugs, thereby reducing dose-related drug toxicity and side effects. In addition, it can reduce the risk of respiratory complications [36, 79-81].

Mathematical modeling showed a reduction in the risk of emergence of resistant strains during early phases of a pandemic with the use of two antivirals compared to single antiviral therapy. Among antivirals that are active against influenza virus, a combination of NA inhibitors is attractive because both compounds are licensed for seasonal influenza, they are delivered to the respiratory tract by distinct means (directly through a disc inhaler for zanamivir and after gastrointestinal absorption and hepatic metabolism for oseltamivir), and key mutations associated with resistance are different for each drug. However, negative interactions cannot be ruled out due to possible competition between these two drugs, which target the same binding pocket in NA [15, 80].

The currently available influenza antivirals have a number of limitations; therefore, more effective antiviral strategies are needed. Drug combination studies *in vitro* and *in vivo* have shown the potential for synergistic or additive antiviral activity and for inhibiting the development of resistance; these qualities must be demonstrated in clinical trials.

The planning of such studies is ongoing, and consideration is being given to clinical and virologic evaluations with a determination of influenza virus loads in the patient, a molecular and biological characterization of viruses for resistance and fitness, and a detailed collection of pharmacokinetic data to evaluate safety and toxicity. All of the available information supports the initiation of clinical trials on combination chemotherapy for influenza. Future considerations for combination therapy are dual NA inhibitors, triple combinations, and the inclusion of novel agents. New strategies directed at unexplored targets, such as drugs that affect host antiviral responses, should also be developed [36].

Conclusion

During both a pandemic and routine seasonal influenza, antiviral medications are used to decrease the duration and severity of a patient's symptoms, and these drugs are more effective if they are taken within 48 hours of symptom presentation. The currently available treatment includes two classes of drugs: inhibitors of the M2 ion channel (amantadine and rimantadine) and NA inhibitors (zanamivir and oseltamivir). An initial analysis showed that the new swine flu strain of influenza A (H1N1) was sensitive to NA inhibitors, such as oseltamivir, zanamivir, peramivir and laninamivir, but resistant to adamantanes.

However, despite the proven efficacy of treatment, increasing cases of viral resistance have been observed. Therefore, the currently available influenza antivirals have a number of limitations, and more effective antiviral strategies are needed.

The possibilities include parenteral NA inhibitors, the development of novel antiviral drugs (polymerase and endonuclease inhibitors, sialidases, long-acting NA inhibitors, hemagglutinin inhibitors, and non-structural protein NS1 inhibitors), and immunotherapy. Combination therapy with two or more drugs is a promising approach for the control of seasonal influenza and severe infection with highly pathogenic H5N1 influenza viruses.

REFERENCES

[1] A. Örtqvist, I. Berggren,M. Insulander, B. de Jong, and B. Svenungsson, "Effectiveness of an adjuvanted monovalent vaccine against the 2009 pandemic strain of influenza A(H1N1)v, in Stockholm county, Sweden," *Clinical Infectious Diseases*, vol.52, no. 10, pp. 1203–1211, 2011.

[2] F. G. Hayden and A. J. Hay, "Emergence and transmission of influenza A viruses resistant to amantadine and rimantadine," *Current Topics in Microbiology and Immunology*, vol. 176, pp.119–130, 1992.

[3] Toshiyuki Hikita, Hiroyuki Hikita, Fusako Hikita, Naoko Hikita, and Shizue Hikita. Clinical Effectiveness of Peramivir in Comparison with Other Neuraminidase Inhibitors in Pediatric Influenza Patients. *International Journal of Pediatrics*, Volume 2012, Article ID 834181, 4 pages.

[4] Anthony E. Fiore, Alicia Fry, David Shay, Larisa Gubareva, Joseph S. Bresee, Timothy M. Uyeki. *Antiviral Agents for the Treatment and Chemoprophylaxis of Influenza*. MMWR / January 21, 2011 / Vol. 60 / No. 1

[5] David Reddy. Responding to pandemic (H1N1) 2009 influenza: the role of oseltamivir. *J. Antimicrob. Chemother* 2010; 65 Suppl 2: ii35–40.

[6] Jain S, Kamimoto L, Bramley AM, et al. Hospitalized patients with 2009 H1N1 influenza in the United States, April–June 2009. *N. Engl. J. Med.* 2009;361:1935–44.

[7] Siston AM, Rasmussen SA, Honein MA, et al. Pandemic 2009 influenza A(H1N1) virus illness among pregnant women in the United States. *JAMA* 2010;303:1517–25.

[8] McGeer A, Green KA, Plevneshi A, et al. Antiviral therapy and outcomes of influenza requiring hospitalization in Ontario, Canada. *Clin. Infect Dis.* 2007;45:1568–75.

[9] Dapat IC, Dapat C, Baranovich T, Suzuki Y, Kondo H, et al. (2012) Genetic Characterization of Human Influenza Viruses in the Pandemic (2009–2010) and Post-Pandemic (2010–2011) Periods in Japan. *PLoS ONE* 7(6): e36455. doi:10.1371/journal.pone.0036455.

[10] CDC. Deaths related to 2009 pandemic influenza A (H1N1) among American Indian/Alaska Natives—12 states, 2009. *MMWR* 2009;58:1341–4.

[11] Jain S, Kamimoto L, Bramley AM, et al. Hospitalized patients with 2009 H1N1 influenza in the United States, April–June 2009. *N. Engl. J. Med.* 2009;361:1935–44.

[12] Louie JK, Acosta M, Winter K, et al. Factors associated with death or hospitalization due to pandemic 2009 influenza A(H1N1) infection in California. *JAMA* 2009;302:1896–902.

[13] Nicholson KG, Aoki FY, Osterhaus AD, Trottier S, Carewicz O, et al. (2000) Efficacy and safety of oseltamivir in treatment of acute influenza: a randomized controlled trial. Neuraminidase Inhibitor Flu Treatment Investigator Group. *Lancet* 355: 1845–1850.

[14] Treanor JJ, Hayden FG, Vrooman PS, Barbarash R, Bettis R, et al. (2000) Efficacy and safety of the oral neuraminidase inhibitor oseltamivir in treating acute influenza: a randomized controlled trial. U.S. Oral Neuraminidase Study Group. *JAMA* 283: 1016–1024.

[15] Duval X, van der Werf S, Blanchon T, Mosnier A, Bouscambert-Duchamp M, et al. (2010) Efficacy of Oseltamivir-Zanamivir Combination Compared to Each Monotherapy for Seasonal Influenza: A Randomized Placebo-Controlled Trial. PLoS Med 7(11): e1000362. doi:10.1371/journal.pmed.1000362.

[16] Anne Moscona. Neuraminidase Inhibitors for Influenza. N. Engl. J. Med. 2005; 353:1363-1373September 29, 2005DOI: 10.1056 /NEJMra 050740.

[17] Jefferson T, Jones M, Doshi P, Del Mar C (2009) Neuraminidase inhibitors for preventing and treating influenza in healthy adults: systematic review and meta-analysis. *BMJ* 339: b5106.

[18] Meindl P, Bodo G, Palese P, Schulman J, Tuppy H. Inhibition of neuraminidase activity by derivatives of 2-deoxy-2,3-dehydro-N-acetylneuraminic acid. *Virology* 1974;58:457-63.

[19] Palese P, Compans RW. Inhibition of influenza virus replication in tissue culture by 2-deoxy-2,3-dehydro-N-trifluoroacetylneuraminic acid (FANA): mechanism of action. *J. Gen. Virol.* 1976;33:159-63.

[20] Palese P, Schulman JL, Bodo G, Meindl P. Inhibition of influenza and parainfluenza virus replication in tissue culture by 2-deoxy-2,3-dehydro-N-trifluoroacetylneuraminic acid (FANA). *Virology* 1974;59:490-8.

[21] Varghese JN, McKimm-Breschkin JL, Caldwell JB, Kortt AA, Colman PM. The structure of the complex between influenza virus neuraminidase and sialic acid, the viral receptor. *Proteins* 1992;14:327-32.

[22] von Itzstein M, Wu W-Y, Kok GB, et al. Rational design of potent sialidase-based inhibitors of influenza virus replication. *Nature* 1993;363:418-23.

[23] Varghese JN, Epa VC, Colman PM. Threedimensional structure of the complex of 4-guanidino-Neu5Ac2en and influenza virus neuraminidase. *Protein Sci.* 1995;4:1081-7.
[24] Roche Laboratories Inc. Tamiflu (oseltamivir phosphate) capsules and oral suspension [package insert]. Nutley, NJ: Roche laboratories, Inc.; 2009.
[25] CDC. Updated Interim Recommendations for the Use of Antiviral Medications in the Treatment and Prevention of Influenza for the 2009–2010 Season. http://www.cdc.gov/h1n1flu/recommendations.htm (22 October 2009, date last accessed).
[26] European Centre for Disease Prevention and Control (ECDC). On Public Health Use of Influenza Antivirals During Influenza Pandemics (With Particular References to the Pandemic (H1N1) 2009). http://www.ecdc.europa.eu/en/healthtopics/Documents/0908_Influenza_AH1N1_On_Public_Health_Use_of_Influenza_Antivirals_during_Influenza_Pandemics.pdf (22 October 2009, date last accessed).
[27] WHO. WHO Guidelines for Parmacological Management of Pandemic (H1N1) 2009 Influenza and Other Influenza Viruses. http://www.who.int/entity/csr/resources/publications/swineflu/h1n1_guidelines_pharmaceutical_mngt.pdf (22 October 2009, date last accessed).
[28] Kim CU, Lew W, Williams MA, et al. Influenza neuraminidase inhibitors possessing a novel hydrophobic interaction in the enzyme active site: design, synthesis, and structural analysis of carbocyclic sialic acid analogues with potent anti-influenza activity. *J. Am. Chem. Soc.* 1997;119:681-90.
[29] Karie S, Launay-Vacher V, Janus N, et al. Pharmacokinetics and dosage adjustment of oseltamivir and zanamivir in patients with renal failure. *Nephrol. Dial Transplant* 2006;21:3606–8.
[30] Burch J, Corbett M, Stock C, Nicholson K, Elliot AJ, et al. (2009) Prescription of anti-influenza drugs for healthy adults: a systematic review and meta-analysis. *Lancet Infect Dis.* 9: 537–545.
[31] Treanor JJ, Hayden FG, Vrooman PS, et al. Efficacy and safety of the oral neuraminidase inhibitor oseltamivir in treating acute influenza: a randomized controlled trial. *JAMA* 2000;283:1016-24.
[32] Aoki FY, Macleod MD, Paggiaro P, et al. Early administration of oral oseltamivir increases the benefits of influenza treatment. *J. Antimicrob. Chemother* 2003;51:123-9.
[33] Hayden FG, Belshe R, Villanueva C, et al. Management of influenza in households: a prospective, randomized comparison of oseltamivir

treatment with or without postexposure prophylaxis. *J. Infect Dis.* 2004;189:440-9.

[34] Oxford J, Balasingam S, Lambkin R. A new millennium conundrum: how to use a powerful class of influenza anti-neuraminidase drugs (NAIs) in the community. *J. Antimicrob. Chemother* 2004;53:133-6.

[35] Ferraris, O.; Lina, B. Mutations of neuraminidase implicated in neuraminidase inhibitors resistance. *J. Clin. Virol.* 2008, 41, 13-19.

[36] Govorkova E.A., Webster R.G. Combination Chemotherapy for Influenza. *Viruses*. 2010; 2(8):1510-1529.

[37] Yen, H-L; Herlocher, L.M.; Hoffmann, E.; Matrosovich, M.N.; Monto, A.S.; Webster. R.G.; Govorkova, E.A. Neuraminidase inhibitor-resistant influenza viruses may differ substantially in fitness and transmissibility. Antimicrob. *Agents Chemother*. 2005, 49, 4075-4084.

[38] Bouvier, N.M.; Lowen, A.C.; Palese, P. Oseltamivir-resistant influenza A viruses are transmitted efficiently among guinea pigs by direct contact but not by aerosol. *J. Virol.* 2008, 82, 10052-10058.

[39] Lackenby, A.; Hungnes, O.; Dudman, S.G.; Meijer, A.; Paget, W.J.; Hay, A. J.; Zambon, M.C. Emergence of resistance to oseltamivir among influenza A (H1N1) viruses in Europe. *Eurosurveillance* 2008, 13, 1–3.

[40] Dharan, N.J.; Gubareva, L.V.; Meyer, J.J.; Okomo-Adhiambo, M.; McClinton, R.C.; Marshall, S.A.; George, K. St.; Epperson, S.; Brammer, L.; Klimov, A.I.; Bresee, J.S.; Fry, A.M. For the Oseltamivir-Resistance Working Group. Infections with oseltamivir-resistant influenza A (H1N1) virus in the United States. *JAMA* 2009, 301, 1034-1041.

[41] Hurt, A.C.; Ernest, J.; Deng, Y-M.; Iannello, P.; Besselaar, T.G.; Birch, C.; Buchy, P.; Chittaganpitch, M.; Chiu, S-C.; Dwyer, D.; Guigoni, A.; Harrower, B.; Kei, I.P.; Kok, T.; Lin, C.; McPhie, K.; Mohd, A.; Olveda, R.; Panayotou, T.; Rawlinson, W.; Scott, L.; Smith, D.; D'Souza, H.; Komadina, N.; Shaw, R.; Kelso, A.; Barr, I.G. Emergence and spread of oseltamivir-resistant A (H1N1) influenza viruses in Oceania, South East Asia and South Africa. *Antiviral Res.* 2009, 83, 90-93.

[42] Baz M, Abed Y, Papenburg J, et al. Emergence of oseltamivir-resistant pandemic H1N1 virus during prophylaxis. *N. Engl. J. Med.* 2009; 361:2296–7.

[43] Le QM, Wertheim HF, Tran ND, et al. A community cluster of oseltamivir-resistant cases of 2009 H1N1 influenza. *N. Engl. J. Med.* 2010;362:86–7.

[44] CDC. Update: influenza activity—United States, 2009–10 season. *MMWR* 2010;59:901–8.

[45] CDC. Oseltamivir-resistant novel influenza A (H1N1) virus infection in two immunosuppressed patients—Seattle, Washington, 2009. *MMWR* 2009;58:893–6.

[46] CDC. Oseltamivir-resistant 2009 pandemic influenza A (H1N1) virus infection in two summer campers receiving prophylaxis—North Carolina, 2009. *MMWR* 2009;58:969–72.

[47] Glaxo Wellcome Inc. Relenza (zanimivir for inhalation) [Package insert]. Research Triangle Park, NC: Glaxo Wellcome, Inc.; 2009.

[48] Cass LM, Efthymiopoulous C, Bye A. Pharmacokinetics of zanamivir after intravenous, oral, inhaled or intranasal administration to healthy volunteers. *Clin. Pharmacokinet* 1999; 36(Suppl 1):1–11.

[49] Hayden F. Developing new antiviral agents for influenza treatment: what does the future hold? *Clin. Infect Dis*. 2009;48(Suppl 1):S3–13.

[50] Calfee DP, Peng AW, Cass LM, Lobo M, Hayden FG. Safety and efficacy of intravenous zanamivir in preventing experimental human influenza A virus infection. *Antimicrob. Agents Chemother* 1999; 43:1616–20.

[51] Gaur AH, Bagga B, Barman S, et al. Intravenous zanamivir for oseltamivir-resistant 2009 H1N1 influenza. *N. Engl. J. Med.* 2010;362:88–9.

[52] Kidd IM, Down J, Nastouli E, et al. H1N1 pneumonitis treated with intravenous zanamivir. *Lancet* 2009;374:1036.

[53] Bautista E, Chotpitayasunondh T, Gao Z, et al. Clinical aspects of pandemic 2009 influenza A (H1N1) virus infection. *N. Engl. J. Med.* 2010;362:1708–19.

[54] Dulek DE, Williams JV, Creech CB, et al. Use of intravenous zanamivir after development of oseltamivir resistance in a critically ill immunosuppressed child infected with 2009 pandemic influenza A (H1N1) virus. *Clin. Infect Dis*. 2010;50:1493–6.

[55] Stittelaar KJ, Tisdale M, van Amerongen G, et al. Evaluation of intravenous zanamivir against experimental influenza A(H5N1) virus infection in the cynomolgus macaques. *Antivir. Res*. 2008; 80:225–8.

[56] Higgs ES, Hayden FG, Chotpitayasunondh T, Whitworth J, Farrar J. The Southeast Asia Influenza Clinical Research Network: development and challenges for a new multilateral research endeavor. *Antivir. Res*. 2008; 78:64–8.

[57] Ison MG, Gnann JW Jr, Nagy-Agren S, et al. Safety and efficacy of nebulized zanamivir in hospitalized patients with serious influenza. *Antivir Ther* 2003;8:183–90.

[58] Kiatboonsri S, Kiatboonsri CTheerawit P. Fatal respiratory events caused by zanamivir nebulization. *Clin. Infect Dis*. 2009;50:620.

[59] LaForce C, Man CY, Henderson FW, et al. Efficacy and safety of inhaled zanamivir in the prevention of influenza in community-dwelling, high-risk adult and adolescent subjects: a 28-day, multicenter, randomized, double-blind, placebo-controlled trial. *Clin. Ther.* 2007;29:1579–90; discussion 1577–8.

[60] Gupta YK, Padhy BM. Issues in pharmacotherapy of 2009 H1N1 influenza infection. *J. Postgrad. Med.* 2010;56:321-7.

[61] Krug RM, Aramini JM. Emerging antiviral targets for influenza A virus. *Trends Pharmacol. Sci.* 2009;30:269–277.

[62] Freund B, Gravenstein S, Elliott M, Miller I. Zanamivir: a review of clinical safety. *Drug Saf.* 1999;21:267-81.

[63] Greer LG, Sheffield JS, Rogers VL, et al. Maternal and neonatal outcomes after antepartum treatment of influenza with antiviral medications. *Obstet. Gynecol.* 2010;115:711–6.

[64] Murphy KR, Eivindson A, Pauksens K, et al. Efficacy and safety of inhaled zanamivir for the treatment of influenza in patients with asthma or chronic obstructive pulmonary disease: a double-blind, randomised, placebo-controlled, multicentre study. *Clin. Drug Investig.* 2000;20:337-49.

[65] Kristian Thorlund, Tahany Awad, Guy Boivin and Lehana Thabane. Systematic review of influenza resistance to the neuraminidase inhibitors. *BMC Infectious Diseases* 2011, 11:134.

[66] Gubareva LV, Kaiser L, Matrosovich MN, et al. Selection of influenza virus mutants in experimentally infected volunteers treated with oseltamivir. *J. Infect Dis.* 2001;183:523–31.

[67] Barnett JM, Cadman A, Gor D, et al. Zanamivir susceptibility monitoring and characterization of influenza virus clinical isolates obtained during phase II clinical efficacy studies. *Antimicrob. Agents Chemother* 2000;44:78–87.

[68] Gubareva LV, Fry AM. Current challenges in the risk assessment of neuraminidase inhibitor-resistant influenza viruses. *J. Infect Dis.* 2010;201:656–8.

[69] Ison MG, Gubareva LV, Atmar RL, et al. Recovery of drug-resistant influenza virus from immunocompromised patients: a case series. *J. Infect Dis.* 2006;193:760–4.

[70] Kohno S, Kida H, Mizuguchi M, Shimada J. Efficacy and safety of intravenous peramivir for treatment of seasonal influenza virus infection. *Antimicrob. Agents Chemother.* 2010 Nov;54(11):4568-74.

[71] Kohno S, Kida H, Mizuguchi M, Hirotsu N, Ishida T, Kadota J, Shimada J. Intravenous peramivir for treatment of influenza A and B virus infection in high-risk patients. *Antimicrob. Agents Chemother.* 2011 Jun;55(6):2803-12.

[72] Shetty AK, Peek LA. Peramivir for the treatment of influenza. *Expert Rev. Anti Infect Ther.* 2012 Feb;10(2):123-43.

[73] Sugaya N, Kohno S, Ishibashi T, Wajima T, Takahashi T. Efficacy, safety, and pharmacokinetics of intravenous peramivir in childrenwith 2009 pandemic H1N1 influenza A virus infection. *Antimicrob. Agents Chemother.* 2012 Jan;56(1):369-77.

[74] Hernandez JE, Adiga R, Armstrong R, Bazan J, Bonilla H, Bradley J, Dretler R, Ison MG, Mangino JE, Maroushek S, Shetty AK, Wald A, Ziebold C, Elder J, Hollister AS, Sheridan W. Clinical experience in adults and children treated with intravenous peramivir for 2009 influenza A (H1N1) under an Emergency IND program in the United States. *Clin. Infect Dis.* 2011 Mar 15;52(6):695-706.

[75] Watanabe, A. A randomized double-blind controlled study of laninamivir compared with oseltamivir for the treatment of influenza in patients with chronic respiratory diseases. *J. Infect Chemother.* 2012 Aug 21. [Epub ahead of print].

[76] Kubo S, Tomozawa T, Kakuta M, Tokumitsu A, Yamashita M. Laninamivir prodrug CS-8958, a long-acting neuraminidase inhibitor, shows superior anti-influenzavirus activity after a single administration. *Antimicrob. Agents Chemother.* 2010 Mar;54(3):1256-64.

[77] Katsumi Y, Otabe O, Matsui F, Kidowaki S, Mibayashi A, Tsuma Y, Ito H. Effect of a single inhalation of laninamivir octanoate in children with influenza. *Pediatrics.* 2012 Jun;129(6):e1431-6.

[78] Vavricka CJ, Li Q, Wu Y, Qi J, Wang M, Liu Y, Gao F, Liu J, Feng E, He J, Wang J, Liu H, Jiang H, Gao GF. Structural and functional analysis of laninamivir and its octanoate prodrug reveals group specific mechanisms for influenza NA inhibition. *PLoS Pathog.* 2011 Oct;7(10):e1002249.

[79] Poland GA, Jacobson RM, Ovsyannikova IG (2009) Influenza virus resistance to antiviral agents: a plea for rational use. *Clin. Infect Dis*. 48: 1254–1256.

[80] Wu JT, Leung GM, Lipsitch M, Cooper BS, Riley S (2009) Hedging against antiviral resistance during the next influenza pandemic using small stockpiles of an alternative chemotherapy. *PLoS Med.* 6: e1000085. doi:10.1371/journal. pmed.1000085.

[81] Sheu TG, Deyde VM, Okomo-Adhiambo M, Garten RJ, Xu X, et al. (2008) Surveillance for neuraminidase inhibitor resistance among human influenza A and B viruses circulating worldwide from 2004 to 2008. *Antimicrob. Agents Chemother* 52: 3284–3292.

treatment with or without postexposure prophylaxis. *J. Infect Dis.* 2004;189:440-9.

[34] Oxford J, Balasingam S, Lambkin R. A new millennium conundrum: how to use a powerful class of influenza anti-neuraminidase drugs (NAIs) in the community. *J. Antimicrob. Chemother* 2004;53:133-6.

[35] Ferraris, O.; Lina, B. Mutations of neuraminidase implicated in neuraminidase inhibitors resistance. *J. Clin. Virol.* 2008, 41, 13-19.

[36] Govorkova E.A., Webster R.G. Combination Chemotherapy for Influenza. *Viruses*. 2010; 2(8):1510-1529.

[37] Yen, H-L; Herlocher, L.M.; Hoffmann, E.; Matrosovich, M.N.; Monto, A.S.; Webster. R.G.; Govorkova, E.A. Neuraminidase inhibitor-resistant influenza viruses may differ substantially in fitness and transmissibility. Antimicrob. *Agents Chemother*. 2005, 49, 4075-4084.

[38] Bouvier, N.M.; Lowen, A.C.; Palese, P. Oseltamivir-resistant influenza A viruses are transmitted efficiently among guinea pigs by direct contact but not by aerosol. *J. Virol.* 2008, 82, 10052-10058.

[39] Lackenby, A.; Hungnes, O.; Dudman, S.G.; Meijer, A.; Paget, W.J.; Hay, A. J.; Zambon, M.C. Emergence of resistance to oseltamivir among influenza A (H1N1) viruses in Europe. *Eurosurveillance* 2008, 13, 1–3.

[40] Dharan, N.J.; Gubareva, L.V.; Meyer, J.J.; Okomo-Adhiambo, M.; McClinton, R.C.; Marshall, S.A.; George, K. St.; Epperson, S.; Brammer, L.; Klimov, A.I.; Bresee, J.S.; Fry, A.M. For the Oseltamivir-Resistance Working Group. Infections with oseltamivir-resistant influenza A (H1N1) virus in the United States. *JAMA* 2009, 301, 1034-1041.

[41] Hurt, A.C.; Ernest, J.; Deng, Y-M.; Iannello, P.; Besselaar, T.G.; Birch, C.; Buchy, P.; Chittaganpitch, M.; Chiu, S-C.; Dwyer, D.; Guigoni, A.; Harrower, B.; Kei, I.P.; Kok, T.; Lin, C.; McPhie, K.; Mohd, A.; Olveda, R.; Panayotou, T.; Rawlinson, W.; Scott, L.; Smith, D.; D'Souza, H.; Komadina, N.; Shaw, R.; Kelso, A.; Barr, I.G. Emergence and spread of oseltamivir-resistant A (H1N1) influenza viruses in Oceania, South East Asia and South Africa. *Antiviral Res.* 2009, 83, 90-93.

[42] Baz M, Abed Y, Papenburg J, et al. Emergence of oseltamivir-resistant pandemic H1N1 virus during prophylaxis. *N. Engl. J. Med.* 2009; 361:2296–7.

[43] Le QM, Wertheim HF, Tran ND, et al. A community cluster of oseltamivir-resistant cases of 2009 H1N1 influenza. *N. Engl. J. Med.* 2010;362:86–7.

[44] CDC. Update: influenza activity—United States, 2009–10 season. *MMWR* 2010;59:901–8.

[45] CDC. Oseltamivir-resistant novel influenza A (H1N1) virus infection in two immunosuppressed patients—Seattle, Washington, 2009. *MMWR* 2009;58:893–6.

[46] CDC. Oseltamivir-resistant 2009 pandemic influenza A (H1N1) virus infection in two summer campers receiving prophylaxis—North Carolina, 2009. *MMWR* 2009;58:969–72.

[47] Glaxo Wellcome Inc. Relenza (zanimivir for inhalation) [Package insert]. Research Triangle Park, NC: Glaxo Wellcome, Inc.; 2009.

[48] Cass LM, Efthymiopoulous C, Bye A. Pharmacokinetics of zanamivir after intravenous, oral, inhaled or intranasal administration to healthy volunteers. *Clin. Pharmacokinet* 1999; 36(Suppl 1):1–11.

[49] Hayden F. Developing new antiviral agents for influenza treatment: what does the future hold? *Clin. Infect Dis*. 2009;48(Suppl 1):S3–13.

[50] Calfee DP, Peng AW, Cass LM, Lobo M, Hayden FG. Safety and efficacy of intravenous zanamivir in preventing experimental human influenza A virus infection. *Antimicrob. Agents Chemother* 1999; 43:1616–20.

[51] Gaur AH, Bagga B, Barman S, et al. Intravenous zanamivir for oseltamivir-resistant 2009 H1N1 influenza. *N. Engl. J. Med.* 2010;362:88–9.

[52] Kidd IM, Down J, Nastouli E, et al. H1N1 pneumonitis treated with intravenous zanamivir. *Lancet* 2009;374:1036.

[53] Bautista E, Chotpitayasunondh T, Gao Z, et al. Clinical aspects of pandemic 2009 influenza A (H1N1) virus infection. *N. Engl. J. Med.* 2010;362:1708–19.

[54] Dulek DE, Williams JV, Creech CB, et al. Use of intravenous zanamivir after development of oseltamivir resistance in a critically ill immunosuppressed child infected with 2009 pandemic influenza A (H1N1) virus. *Clin. Infect Dis*. 2010;50:1493–6.

[55] Stittelaar KJ, Tisdale M, van Amerongen G, et al. Evaluation of intravenous zanamivir against experimental influenza A(H5N1) virus infection in the cynomolgus macaques. *Antivir. Res.* 2008; 80:225–8.

[56] Higgs ES, Hayden FG, Chotpitayasunondh T, Whitworth J, Farrar J. The Southeast Asia Influenza Clinical Research Network: development and challenges for a new multilateral research endeavor. *Antivir. Res.* 2008; 78:64–8.

In: Swine Flu
Editors: J. C. Marie and T. B. Johnson ISBN: 978-1-62618-363-6

Chapter 2

Epidemiology and Recent Topics Regarding Swine Flu in Adults: After the 2009 Flu Pandemic

Nobuhiro Asai
Department of Pulmonology, Kameda Medical Center, Chiba, Japan

Abstract

Influenza is one of the most common infections worldwide. It often causes a life-threatening illness in humans. The pandemic of 2009 is still fresh in our memory.

While a large amount of information concerning the natural history and clinical management of 2009 H1N1 virus infection has been obtained in a remarkably short period, there are several medical problems still remaining.

They are; analyzing risk factors among patients with swine flu for severe illness, the effectiveness of vaccination, the management for swine flu and its complications, the emergence of oseltamivir-resistant influenza virus and therapeutic options such as extracorporeal membrane oxygenation (ECMO) and traditional herbal medicine.

This article describes the epidemiology, clinical manifestations, risk factors, preventive methods, treatment options and new topics on swine flu.

INTRODUCTION

During the spring of 2009, a novel influenza A (H1N1) virus of swine origin caused human infection resulting in acute respiratory illness in Mexico [1, 2]. After initially spreading by human to human transmission in the United States and Canada [3, 4], the virus spread globally, resulting in the first influenza pandemic in the 21 century since 1968. Finally, the World Health Organization (WHO) raised the influenza pandemic alert to phase 6, which is the highest level [5]. As of March 2010, almost all countries had reported cases, and more than 17,700 deaths among laboratory-confirmed cases were reported to the WHO [6].

The H1N1 influenza is a novel strain of the influenza A virus and is widely known as swine flu. The virus contains a mixture of genetic material from human, pig and bird flu virus. It is a new variety of flu which people have not had much immunity to [1, 2]. The influenza A virus has been responsible for three previous global pandemics; Spanish flu in 1918 [7, 8], Asian flu in 1957 [8, 9] and Hong Kong flu in 1968 [8, 9]. The 1918 pandemic, what we called Spanish flu, is the most severe pandemic which caused severe pneumonia. It was estimated that 20 to 40 million people died globally in the 1918 pandemic [7, 8] (Table 1). The severity of the 2009 pandemic is thought to be similar to the one of the Spanish flu. Like seasonal influenza, the virus of this influenza pandemic appeared primarily to affect children, young adults and pregnant woman, as well as those with underlying conditions. It is striking that 25 to 50% of patients who were hospitalized or died had no comorbidity [10].

Table 1. Comparison of previous pandemics between in the 20th and 21st century

Pandemic	Spanish flu in 1918	Asian flu in 1957	Hong Kong flu in 1968	The pandemic in 2009
Strain	A (H1N1)	A (H2N2)	A (H3N2)	A (H1N1)
Year	1918-1919	1957-1958	1968-1969	2009-2010
Origin	Not known	China	China	Mexico
Estimated global death	20 to 40 million	1 million	1 to 4 million	17,700
Groups most affected	20 to 40 years	School children and elderly	Elderly	5 to 65 years

A previous report suggested that 33% of individuals over 60 years of age had neutralizing antibodies to A/California/04/09, likely due to previous exposure to antigenically similar H1N1 viruses [11].

It is reasonable that younger patients without any underlying disease who had no immunity to the 2009 (H1N1) influenza virus got worse, resulting in death.

While a large amount of information concerning the natural history and clinical management of 2009 H1N1 virus infection has been obtained in a remarkably short period, there are several medical problems still remaining such as the occurrence of multi-drugs-resistant virus [12], treatments for complications or the efficacy of vaccination [13, 14]. This article describes the history and recent topics about swine flu.

VIRAL CHARACTERISTICS

Triple-reassortant swine influenza viruses, including genes from human, swine, and avian influenza A viruses, have been identified in swine in the United States since 1998 [15, 16], and 12 cases of human infection with such viruses were identified in the United States from 2005 through 2009 [17].

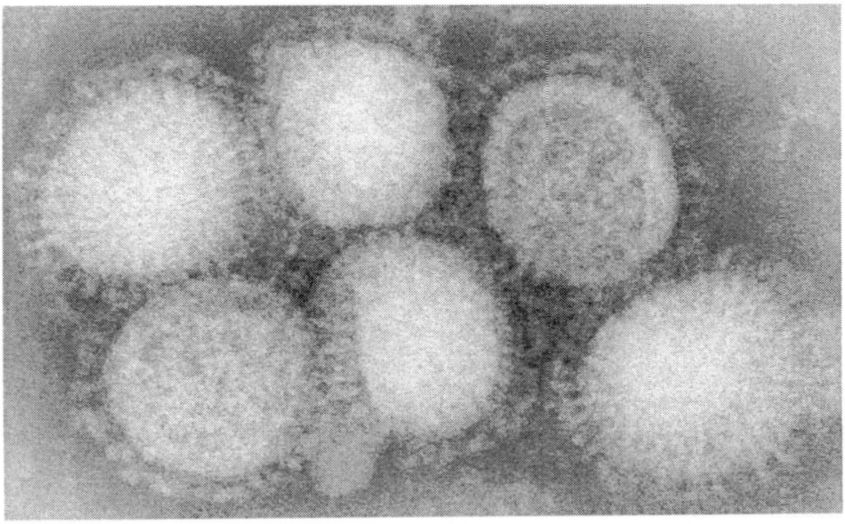

Cited by Wikipedia.

Figure 1. Influenza virus by electron microscope.

A novel swine-origin influenza A (H1N1) was identified and in June 2009 [18], WHO declared the new strain of swine-origin H1N1 as a pandemic. This strain of virus is often called as swine flu by the public media. After initially spreading among people in Mexico and Canada, the virus spread rapidly and globally, resulting in the pandemic 2009 [18]. The 2009 H1N1 virus derives six genes from triple-reassortant North American swine flu virus lineages and two genes from Eurasian swine virus lineages. Although the 2009 H1N1 virus is antigenically distinct from other human and swine influenza A (H1N1) viruses, strains of this virus is antigenically homogenous [4]. Some reported that the level of pulmonary replication of the 2009 H1N1 virus is higher than that of seasonal influenza A viruses in experimentally infected animals [11, 19, 20].

Studies of hemagglutinin-receptor binding indicate that the 2009 H1N1 virus is well adapted to mammalian hosts and binds to both α2,6-linked cellular receptors and α2,3-linked recptors, which are present in the conjunctivae, distal airway and alveolar pneumocytes [21]. The 2009 H1N1 virus shows increased ex vivo replication in human bronchial epithelium at 33^{0}C, as compared with a seasonal influenza virus [22]. It is also characterized by increased replication and pathological changes in the lungs of nonhuman primates and increased replication in ex vivo human tissues [11]. These might help explain the ability of the virus to cause severe viral pneumonitis in patients infected with the 2009 H1N1 virus.

Clinical Presentation

Signs and Symptoms

Most patients present typical influenza-like illness such as fever, dry cough, headache, muscle or joint pain, sore throat, chills, fatigue, and runny nose [2, 23-25]. While fever is the most common symptom, mild illness without fever has been reported in 8 to 32% of infected persons [26]. Diarrhea, vomiting, and neurological problems have also been reported in some cases. Notably, gastrointestinal symptoms are more frequent than seasonal influenza in adult.

Dyspnea, tachycardia in children, chest pain, purulent sputum, prolonged or recurrent fever, altered mental status, dehydration, and reappearance of lower respiratory symptoms after improvement are signs of progression to more severe disease or complications [2, 27-29].

Complications

Infection with swine flu (H1N1) varies a broad spectrum of clinical syndromes, ranging from afebrile upper respiratory illness to fulminant viral pneumonia [24]. The principal clinical syndrome resulting in hospitalization and intensive care is viral pneumonitis associated with severe hypoxia, acute lung injury (ALI) /acute respiratory distress syndrome (ARDS), and multiple organ failure (MOF) [28, 29]. This syndrome has accounted for 49 to 72% of intensive care unit (ICU) admissions for the 2009 H1N1 virus infection. It commonly shows a rapid progression, typically starting on day 4 to 5 after the onset of illness [22, 28, 29]. Intubation and mechanical ventilation is often needed within 24 hours after admission. As for radiological findings, diffuse mixed interstitial and alveolar infiltrates are found on chest computed tomography (CT). On early phase of the illness, it is difficult to find an abnormal shadow on chest X-ray. Thus, clinician must recognize the possibility of this syndrome and chest CT should be performed if influenza pneumonitis is suspected.

Viral infections can cause asthma exacerbation [30, 31]. In particular, influenza virus infections sometimes result in severe respiratory failure [30, 31]. As for patients with chronic obstructive pulmonary disease (COPD), it is well known that the infections can cause acute exacerbation of COPD. Among hospitalized patients with 2009 H1N1 infection, a history of asthma has been reported 24 to 50% of children and adults, and COPD in 36% of adults [32, 33].

Secondary bacterial pneumonia occurs later in the course of illness when viral shedding may have ceased. *Streptococcus pneumonia* is the most common pathogens, followed by *S pyogenes* and *Staphylococcus aureus* [34, 35]. The mechanisms by which influenza increases the risk of contracting severe bacterial infection are still controversial. Some researchers have suggested that influenza may cause viral immunosuppression. An altered cytokine response may strip sialic acid from the lung, thus exposing receptors for bacterial adherence. Early treatment with neuraminidase inhibitors could interrupt the cleavage of sialic acids, resulting in inhibition of this infection [34]. It is well known that bacterial coinfection with influenza A (H1N1) shows a high mortality. Clinicians should consider early coverage for both influenza A (H1N1) and bacterial coinfection in critically ill patients suspected to have influenza.

In terms of extrapulmonary complications of influenza A (H1N1), myocarditis and encephalitis have sporadically been reported [31,36,37]. The number of patients with asymptomatic myocarditis caused by influenza virus might be underdiagnosed. Hemophagocytic syndrome (HPS) could occur more frequently in patients with swine flu than in those with seasonal flu [38,39]. Some documented that HPS would be a risk factor of death, however, it is still controversial [38]. More cases should be estimated and investigated.

Risk Groups and Risk Factors for Severe Disease

While appropriately 25 to 50% of patients with influenza A (H1N1) virus infection who were hospitalized or died had no reported comorbidity, underlying disease or conditions which are associated with complications from seasonal influenza are also risk factors for complications with influenza A (H1N1) virus infection as shown in Table 2.

Note that 33% of individuals over 60 years of age had neutralizing antibodies to A/California/04/09, likely due to previous exposure to antigenically similar H1N1 viruses [22].

Table 2. Risk factors for complications or severe illness with influenza A (H1N1) virus

Risk factors	
Age	<5 or ≧65 years old
Pregnancy	Highest risk in the third trimester
Smoking	Suggested, but not proven to be an independent factor
Obesity	BMI≧35
Chronic heart disease	Congestive heart failure or atherosclerotic disease
Chronic pulmonary disease	Asthma or COPD, cystic fibrosis
Chronic renal disease	Renal dialysis or transplantation
Chronic hepatic disease	Cirrhosis
Immunosuppression	HIV infections or AIDS, diabetes mellitus, malnutrition, organ transplantation, receipt of chemotherapy or corticosteroid or immunosuppressant

* COPD; chronic obstructive pulmonary disease, HIV; human immunodeficiency virus, AIDS; acquired immunodeficiency syndrome.

It is reasonable that patients who had no immunity to the 2009 (H1N1) influenza virus got worse, resulting in death. An epidemiological study about cohorts estimated that the individuals born in and around the pandemic had a 20% excess cardiovascular disease at 60–82 years of age, relative to those born without exposure to the influenza epidemic, thus suggesting that prenatal exposure to even uncomplicated maternal influenza may have lasting consequences later in life [40].

There appeared to be a particularly increased risk factor of death among pregnant women and severe obese patients. During the 2009 influenza pandemic, pregnant women accounted for up to 7–10% of hospitalized patients [24, 32, 33], 6–9% of ICU patients [24, 29, 41] and 6–10% of patients who died [24, 32], compared to 1–2% of pregnancies among a healthy population. This is also consistent with influenza-associated excess deaths among pregnant women during the pandemics of 1917–1918 and 1957–1958 [42].

Louie, et al. documented that severe obesity could be a risk factor among patients with influenza A (H1N1) virus infection [32]. They reported that body mass index (BMI) $\geqq$35 is a risk factor in California, in the United States. I guess that BMI $\geqq$25 to 30 would be a risk factor for complications in Asian populations as our cases show [39]. Too much of cytokines released by lipoma might be associated with development of influenza pneumonitis, resulting in ALI/ ARDS [43, 44].

It is thought that smoking, alcoholism and comorbidities as shown in Table 2 are risk factors among patients with severe or fatal influenza A (H1N1) virus infection [29]. Zarychanski, et al demonstrated that aboriginal status, the presence of coexisting conditions, and delayed receipt of antiviral therapy could independently correlate with severe or fatal cases of influenza A (H1N1) virus infection [43].

DIAGNOSIS

Diagnosis as influenza virus infection is based on influenza like illness during a recognized outbreak. Conventional rapid influenza diagnostic tests (RIDT) had poor clinical sensitivity (11 to 70%) for the detection of the 2009 H1N1 virus in respiratory specimens [46]. The negative test results should not be used to make decisions pending antiviral therapy. Clinical symptoms of influenza A (H1N1) that overlap with those of other common infections have led to the misdiagnosis of other potentially treatable infections [47].

Reverse transcription-PCR tests for the detection of 2009 H1N1 virus were developed by CDC and distributed to state public health and other reference laboratories. Its cost-effectiveness is not good enough to exceed a RIDT [48].

PREVENTIVE METHODS

Vaccine

Influenza vaccination is widely performed. Its efficacy has been discussed for several years. In Japan, the vaccination of schoolchildren was discontinued in 1990s because of doubt about its effectiveness. As a result, excess mortality rates followed among the elderly and children in Japan [48,49]. Likewise, Kawai et al. documented that the mass influenza vaccination of schoolchildren was effective in reducing the number of class cancellation days and absenteeism at school [50]. The Advisory Committee on Immunization Practices (ACIP) recommended that all the students in primary and secondary school should receive influenza vaccine, resulting in prevention of spreading influenza to their family and community [51].

Efficacy and safety of H1N1 vaccine has been reported for seasonal influenza vaccines [52]. However, the immunization rate is still below that recommended. Then, the cost-effectiveness is controversial. Evidence of influenza vaccine for protection in adults aged 65 years or older is lacking. Although several problems about influenza vaccine exist, it remains to be one of the most useful preventive tools for influenza infection among all aged people.

Route of Influenza Transmission

Like seasonal influenza, prevention is as important as treatment. Transmission of swine flu should be the same as for seasonal flu. Influenza is thought to spread mainly by contagion or by droplet infection [53]. However, in mice and ferrets, airborne transmission of influenza virus was already confirmed [54, 55]. Likewise, William et al [56] reported that aerosol particles released by influenza patients are small enough to become an airborne transmission route. Aerosol particle from human cough could be one of routes of influenza transmission. Basic prevention such as gargling, washing, surgical mask and cough etiquette has limited effectiveness to prevent spread of influenza virus. Isolation of influenza patients with cough is important for prevention of airborne transmission.

Post-Exposure Chemoprophylaxis

In randomized, placebo-controlled trials, both oseltamivir and zanamivir were effective in preventing influenza infection among persons receiving chemoprophylaxis after a household member or other close contact had laboratory-confirmed influenza [57, 58]. In addition, a recent report demonstrated that prophylactic neuraminidase inhibitors were effective in a pediatric ward [59]. CDC/IDSA guideline recommended that post-exposure chemoprophylaxis by neuraminidase inhibitors should be used in nursing homes [51]. However, the preventing measure is not commonly performed in Japanese nursing homes, since neuraminidase inhibitors are costly. Japanese nursing homes are managed as comprehensive medical care systems. Due to the medical cost of a nursing home and its system, it is difficult to do chemoprophylaxis.

Temporary Closing of School Classes

The number of patients with influenza is increasing and temporary closing of classes is often seen. While there are some problems such as burden for the family who care for flu patients and delay of education, temporary closing of classes due to flu is effective for prevention of spread and reduction in the number of patients [60].

Treatment

Antiviral Therapy

Neuraminidase inhibitors such as oseltamivir, zanamivir and peramivir are the first choice in the treatment of swine flu (H1N1) infection as well as seasonal influenza virus infection [61, 62]. The 2009 H1N1 virus is generally susceptible to oseltamivir and zanamivir [11, 18]. However, it is mostly resistant to amantadine and rimantadine. The therapy with a neuraminidase inhibitor is very important for high risk group patients (Table 1).

Early therapy with oseltamivir in patients with swine flu (H1N1) virus infection may reduce the duration of hospitalization and the risk of progression to severe disease requiring ICU admission or resulting in death [33,41]. Comparing the death rate in each country in the 2009 pandemic, the death rate in Japan is extremely low as shown in Table 3. In Japan, it is common that physicians prescribe an antiviral drug if influenza infection is suspected. As a result, early treatment for flu could lead to low mortality. In contrast, it has been reported that most patients who died in USA or Mexico visited a health care facility one week after the symptoms were started. These patients' delay could result in high mortality in these countries [63].

It is thought that antiviral therapy for influenza virus infection is useful only when it is used within 48 hours after onset of illness. Even after an interval of more than 48 hours since the onset of illness, however, patients should be treated empirically: it could result in reducing the rate of death among hospitalized patients infected with swine flu (H1N1) virus [16]. As for the treatment for pregnant women with the 2009 H1N1 flu, neuraminidase inhibitors are recommended. In the United Kingdom (UK), zanamivir is the first line treatment of swine flu for pregnant women [63], since zanamivir acts within the respiratory tracts with no absorption into the blood stream. If pregnant patients are not tolerable to inhale the drug due to severe asthma or are hospitalized with complications such as pneumonia, oseltamivir is recommended. Although oseltamivir has been shown to cross the placenta and appears in breast milk, no adverse effects on the fetus or on pregnancy have been recorded [63]. Efficacy and safety of peramivir, which is an intravenous neuraminidase inhibitor in the treatment for pregnant women with swine flu is not established yet.

Table 3. Comparison of death rate in each country in the 2009 pandemic

	USA	Canada	Mexico	Aus	UK	France	NZ	Japan
Number of death	12,000	429	1,111	191	457	309	20	198
Death rate	3.96	1.32	1.05	0.95	0.76	0.50	0.48	0.15

* USA, United States of America; Aus, Australia; UK, United Kingdam; NZ, New Zealand.

Laninamivir is a long-acting neuraminidase inhibitor. A randomized control trial showed its efficacy that is similar to that of oseltamivir in the treatment of seasonal flu as well as oseltamivir-resistant influenza virus [61]. The specialty of this drug is a good compliance. Once inhalation is enough to keep anti-viral effect comparable to that of zanamivir for 5 days inhalation. This drug also would be effective for the 2009 H1N1 influenza virus. Being an inhaler like zanamivir requires some technique, therefore a little child would have difficulty in using this drug [61].

Since the outbreak of influenza A (H1N1) virus pandemic, WHO reported that oseltamivir-resistant influenza virus spread globally as of June 2010 [64]. Peramivir, which is an intravenous neuraminidase inhibitor, provides rapid drug delivery at high levels [23]. The efficacy of peramivir appeared to be similar to that of oseltamivir in adults [66] and peramivir is less active for oseltamivir-resistant influenza viruses carrying the Histidine-to-tyrosine substitution at position 275 (H275Y) than for oseltamivir-susceptible viruses [67, 68]. These strains are typically susceptible to zanamivir. Therefore, intravenous zanamivir is a preferred treatment option for hospitalized patients with suspected or documented oseltamivir-resistant 2009 H1N1 virus infection [3, 68].

ECMO

For patients with the 2009 H1N1 influenza virus-related ARDS, some demonstrated that extracorporeal membrane oxygenation (ECMO) contributes to the low mortality [69, 70]. While it is difficult to evaluate its efficacy by randomized trial because of the difficulty in setting the control group. ECMO would be one of useful tools in the treatment of ARDS patients with influenza pneumonia.

Kampo Medicine

Recently, the efficacy and safety of herbal medicine, which is called kampo medicine for influenza viruses has been reported [71, 72]. On the model of mice infected with influenza virus, some elements act both in anti-inflammatory and in anti-viral effects for influenza virus [73, 74]. Kampo medicine is more economical than neuraminidase inhibiters: its cost is one-half to one-third of antiviral drugs.

Table 4. The component drugs of 8.75g of Saikatsugeki-to

Gypsum	6.0g
Pueraria root	4.0g
Bupleurum root	3.5g
Pinellia tuber	2.5g
Ephedra herb	4.0g
Scutellaria root	1.0g
Cinnamon bark	3.0g
Peony root	3.0g
Glycyrrhiza	3.3g
Ginger	1.7g

4.48g of spray-dried powder extract from these herbs is included in 8.75g of Saikatsugeki-to.

In addition, an adverse effects associated with kampo medicine occurs less frequently than those with oseltamivir. Emergence of a multidrug-resistant influenza A (H1N1) virus has become problematic [75]. Kampo medicine could be one of the useful tools for neuraminidase-resistant influenza infections.

During the pandemic of Spanish flu, the number of fatal flu patients was fewer in Japan than in any other countries. In the pandemic, it is known that saikatsugeki-to (Table 3), which is a kampo medicine commonly used for common cold, contributed to improve the patients with flu. We also conducted a prospective study comparing three groups as follows; oseltamivir alone, oseltamivir plus mao-to and oseltamivr plus saikatsugeki-to Saikatatsugeki-to group showed the efficacy of antipyretic effect and improvement in influenza symptoms. There were no significant differences in the frequency of adverse effects in three groups. More cases should be collected and examined to establish the evidence of kampo medicine in the treatment of influenza virus infection.

CONCLUSION

Although we experienced the first pandemic in the 21th century and amount of information were collected in a very short period, many clinical issues still remain problematic. Alternative ways replacing vaccines should be developed for allergic patients to eggs. While the effectiveness of post-exposure prophylaxis is confirmed, it is difficult to perform it due to economical problem in nursing homes. Flu measure should be aimed for the entire community, globally if possible. Combination of strict hygiene measures, vaccines, post-exposure chemoprophylaxis and early treatment should be the most effective for seasonal as well as swine flu.

ACKNOWLEDGMENT

We are grateful for the diligent and thorough critical reading of our manuscript by Dr. Yoshihiro Ohkuni, the Department of Pulmonology and Mr. John Wocher, Executive Vice President and Director, International Affairs/International Patient Services, Kameda Medical Center (Japan).

REFERENCES

[1] Zuno S, Mejia-Arangure JM, Mar-Obeso AJ, et al. Infection and death from influenza A H1N1 virus in Mexico: a retrospective analysis. *Lancet* 2009; 374:2072-9.

[2] Perez-Padilla R, de la Rosa-Zamboni D, Ponce de Leon S, et al. Pneumonia and respiratory failure from swine-origin influenza A (H1N1) in Mexico. *N. Engl. J. Med.* 2009;361:680-9.

[3] Novel Swine-Origin Influenza A (H1N1) Virus Investigation Team. Emergence of a novel swine-origin influenza A (H1N1) virus in humans. N Engl J Med 2009;360:2605-15. [Erratum, *N. Engl. J. Med.* 2009; 361:102.]

[4] Garten RJ, Davis CT, Russell CA, et al. Antigenic and genetic characteristics of swine-origin 2009 A(H1N1) influenza viruses circulating in humans. *Science* 2009;325:197-201.

[5] Chen M. *World now at the start of 2009 influenza pandemic*. World Health Organization (WHO). 2009. http://www.who.int/ mediacentre/ news/statements/2009/h1n1_pandemic_phase6_20090611/en/index. html.

[6] Pandemic (H1N1) 2009 — update 94. Geneva: World Health Organization, April 1, 2010. (Accessed April 9, 2010, at http://www.who.int/csr/don/2010_04_01/en/index.html.).

[7] Simonsen L, Clarke MJ, Schonberger LB, et al. Pandemic versus epidemic influenza mortality: a pattern of changing age distribution. *J. Infect. Dis.* 1998; 178:53-60.

[8] Luk J, Gross P, Thompson WW. Observations on mortality during the 1918 influenza pandemic. *Clin. Infect. Dis.* 2001; 33:1375-8.

[9] Glezen WP. Emerging infections: pandemic influenza. *Epidemiol. Rev.* 1996; 18:64-76.

[10] Tokimatu I, Kadota J. Serious illness and complications of a new strain of influenza. *kokyukinaika* 2010;17:29-36. Japanese.

[11] Itoh Y, Shinya K, Kiso M, et al. In vitro and in vivo characterization of new swineorigin H1N1 influenza viruses. *Nature* 2009;460:1021-5.

[12] Van der Vries E, Stelma FF, Boucher CA. Emergence of a multidrug-resistant pandemic influenza A (H1N1) virus. *N. Engl. J. Med.* 2010; 363:1381-2.

[13] Zhu FC, Wang H, Fang HH, et al. A novel influenza A (H1N1) vaccine in various age groups. *N. Engl. J. Med.* 2009; 361:2414-23.

[14] Wu J, Xu F, Lu L, et al. Safety and effectiveness of a 2009 H1N1 vaccine in Beijing. *N. Engl. J. Med.* 2010; 363:2416-23.

[15] Olsen CW. The emergence of novel swine influenza viruses in North America. *Virus Res.* 2002; 85:199-210.

[16] Vincent AL, Ma W, Lager KM, Janke BH, Richt JA. Swine influenza viruses:a North American perspective. *Adv. Virus. Res.* 2008; 72:127-54.

[17] Shinde V, Bridges CB, Uyeki TM, et al. Triple-reassortant swine influenza A (H1) in humans in the United States, 2005–2009. *N. Engl. J. Med.* 2009; 360:2616-25.

[18] Novel Swine-Origin Influenza A (H1N1) Virus Investigation Team, Dawood FS, Jain S, Finelli L, et al. Emergence of a novel swine-origin influenza A (H1N1) virus in humans. *N. Engl. J. Med.* 2009; 360: 2605-15.

[19] Maines TR, Jayaraman A, Belser JA, et al. Transmission and pathogenesis of swine-origin 2009 A (H1N1) influenza viruses in ferrets and mice. *Science* 2009;325:484-7.

[20] Munster VJ, de Wit E, van den Brand JM, et al. Pathogenesis and transmission of swine-origin 2009 A (H1N1) influenza virus in ferrets. *Science* 2009; 325:481-3.

[21] Childs RA, Palma AS, Wharton S, et al. Receptor-binding specificity of pandemic influenza A (H1N1) 2009 virus determined by carbohydrate microarray. *Nat. Biotechnol.* 2009; 27:797-9.

[22] Chan MC, Chan RW, Yu WC, et al.Tropism and innate host responses of the 2009 pandemic H1N1 influenza virus in ex vivo and in vitro cultures of humanconjunctiva and respiratory tract. *Am. J. Pathol.* 2010; 176:1828-40.

[23] Writing Committee of the WHO Consultation on Clinical Aspects of Pandemic (H1N1) 2009 Influenza. Clinical Aspects of Pandemic 2009 Influenza A (H1N1) Virus Infection. *N. Engl. J. Med.*2010;362:1708-19.

[24] Poeppl W, Hell M, Herkner H, et al. Clinical aspects of 2009 pandemic influenza A (H1N1) virus infection in Austria. *Infection* 2011;39 341-52.

[25] Takayama K, Kuramochi J, Oinuma T, et al. Clinical features of the 2009 swine-origin influenza A (H1N1) outbreak in Japan. *J Infect. Chemother.* 2011; 17:401-6.

[26] Cao B, Li XW, Mao Y, et al. Clinical features of the initial cases of 2009 pandemic influenza A (H1N1) virus infection in China. *N. Engl. J. Med.* 2009; 361:2507-17.

[27] Dominguez-Cherit G, Lapinsky SE, Macias AE, et al. Critically Ill patients with 2009 influenza A(H1N1) in Mexico. *JAMA* 2009; 302: 1880-7.

[28] The ANZIC Influenza Investigators. Critical care services and 2009 H1N1 influenza in Australia and New Zealand. *N. Engl. J. Med.* 2009; 361:1925-34.

[29] Kumar A, Zarychanski R, Pinto R, et al. Critically ill patients with 2009 influenza A(H1N1) infection in Canada. *JAMA* 2009;302:1872-9.

[30] Cohen L, Castro M. The role of viral respiratory infections in the pathogenesis and exacerbation of asthma. *Semin. Respir. Infect.* 2003; 18:3.

[31] Asai N, Ohkuni Y, Komatsu A, Matsunuma R, Nakashima K, Ando K, et al. A case of asthma complicated influenza myocarditis. *J. Infect. Chemother* 2010; 10:13.

[32] Louie JK, Acosta M, Winter K, et al. Factors associated with 2009 influenza A (H1N1) infection in California. *JAMA* 2009; 302:1896-902.

[33] Jain S, Kamimoto L, Bramley AM, et al. Hospitalized patients with 2009 H1N1 influenza in the United States, April-June 2009. *N. Engl. J. Med.* 2009; 361:1935-44.

[34] Jean C, Louie JK, Glaser CA, et al. Invasive group A streptococcal infection concurrent with 2009 H1N1 influenza. *Clin. Infect. Dis.* 2010; 50:e59-62.

[35] Centers for Disease Control and Prevention (CDC). Bacterial coinfections in lung tissue specimens from fatal cases of 2009 pandemic

influenza A (H1N1) - United States, May-August 2009. *MMWR Morb. Mortal Wkly. Rep.* 2009;58:1071-4.

[36] Noriega LM, Verdugo RJ, Araos R, et al. Pandemic influenza A (H1N1) 2009 with neurological manifestations, a case series. *Influenza Other Respir. Viruses* 2010 Feburary 24 (Epub ahead of print).

[37] Larcombre PJ, Moloney SE, Schmidt PA. Pandemic (H1N1) 2009; a clinical spectrum in the general paediatric population. *Arch. Dis. Child.* 2009 November 10 (Epub ahead of print).

[38] Beutel G, Wiesner O, Eder M, Hafer C, Schneider AS, Kielstein JT, et al. Virus-associated hemophagocytic syndrome as a major contributor to death in patients with 2009 influenza A (H1N1) infection. *Crit. Care.* 2011; 5(2):R80. Epub ahead of print.

[39] Asai N, Ohkuni Y, Matsunuma R, Iwama K, Otsuka Y, Kawamura Y, et al. A case of novel swine influenza A (H1N1) pneumonia complicated with virus-associated hemophagocytic syndrome. *J. Infect. Chemother.* 2012 (Epub ahead of print).

[40] Mazumder B, Almond D, Park K, et al. Lingering prenatal effects of the 1918 influenza pandemic on cardiovascular disease. *J. Dev. Orig. Health Dis.* 2009;10:1–9. doi:10.1017/s2040174409990031.

[41] Louie JK, Acosta M, Jamieson DJ, Honein MA. Severe 2009 H1N1 influenza in pregnant and postpartum women in California. *N. Engl. J. Med.* 2010;362:27–35.

[42] Jamieson DJ, Honein MA, Rasmussen SA, et al. H1N1 2009 influenza virus infection during pregnancy in the USA. *Lancet.* 2009; 374: 451–8.

[43] Gilbert CA, Slingerland JM. Cytokines, Obesity, and Cancer: New Insights on Mechanisms Linking Obesity to Cancer Risk and Progression. *Annu. Rev. Med.* 2012 Oct 26. [Epub ahead of print].

[44] Winfield RD, Delano MJ, Cuenca AG, et al. Obese patients show a depressed cytokine profile following severe blunt injury. *Shock* 2012 Mar; 37(3):253-6.

[45] Zarychanski R, Stuart TL, Kumar A, et al. Correlates of severe disease in patients with 2009 pandemic influenza (H1N1) virus infection. *CMAJ* 2010; 182:257-64.

[46] Clinical management of human infection with pandemic (H1N1) 2009: revised guidance. Geneva: World Health Organization, November 2009. (Accessed April 9, 2010, at http://www.who.int/csr/resource/publications/swineflu/clinical_management/en/index.html.).

[47] Blyth CC, Iredell JR, Dwyer DE. Rapid-test sensitivity for novel swine-origin influenza A (H1N1) virus in humans. *N. Engl. J. Med.* 2009; 361: 2493.

[48] Fiore AE, Fry A, Shay D, Gubareva L, et al. Antiviral agents for the treatment and chemoprophylaxis of influenza --- recommendations of the Advisory Committee on Immunization Practices (ACIP). *MMWR Recomm. Rep.* 2011;60:1-24.

[49] Reichert TA, Sugaya N, Fedson DS, et al. The Japanese experience with vaccinating schoolchildren against influenza. *N. Engl. J. Med.* 2001; 344: 889-96.

[50] Kawai S, Nanri S, Ban E, et al. Influenza vaccination of schoolchildren and influenza outbreaks in a school. *Clin. Infect. Dis.* 2011; 53:130-6.

[51] Fiore AE, Uyeki TM, Broder K, et al. Prevention and control of influenza with vaccines: recommendations of the Advisory Committee on Immunization Practices (ACIP), 2010. *MMWR Recomm. Rep.* 2010; 59(RR-8):1-62.

[52] Zhu FC, Wang H, Fang HH, et al. A novel influenza A (H1N1) vaccine in various age groups. *N. Engl. J. Med.* 2009; 361:2414-23.

[53] Hayden FG, Atmar RL, Schilling M, et al. Use of the selective oral neuraminidase inhibitor oseltamivir to prevent influenza. *N. Engl. J. Med.* 1999;341:1336-43.

[54] Hayden FG, Gubareva LV, Monto AS, et al. Inhaled zanamivir for the prevention of influenza in families. Zanamivir Family Study Group. *N. Engl. J. Med.* 2000;343:1282-9.

[55] Shinjoh M, Takano Y, Takahashi T, et al. Postexposure prophylaxis for influenza in pediatric wards oseltamivir or zanamivir after rapid antigen detection. *Pediatr. Infect. Dis. J.* 2012; 11:1119-23.

[56] Tellier R. Review of aerosol transmission *Emerg. Infect. Dis.* 2006;12:1657-62.

[57] Schulman JL, Kilbourne ED. Airborne transmission *Nature* 1962;195:1129-30.

[58] MacInnes H, Zhou Y, Gouveia K, et al. Transmission of aerosolized seasonal H1N1 influenza *PLoS One* 2011;9:e24448.

[59] Andrewes CH, Lindsley WG, Blachere FM, Thewlis RE, et al. Measurements of airborne influenza virus in aerosol particles from human coughs. *PLoS One* 2010;5:e15100.

[60] Pathogenic microbe detection information. *Pandemic influenza task team.* http://idsc.nih.go.jp/iasr/31/367/dj3671.html.

[61] Moscona A. Neuraminidase inhibitors for influenza. *N. Engl. J. Med.* 2005; 353:1363-73.
[62] Lim BH, Mahmood TA. Influenza A (H1N1) 2009 (Swine flu) and pregnancy. *J. Obstet. Gynaecol. India* 2011; 4:386-93.
[63] Watanabe A, Chang SC, Kim MJ, et al. Long-acting neuraminidase inhibitor laninamivir octanoate versus oseltamivir for treatment of influenza: A double-blind, randomized, noninferiority clinical trial. *Clin. Infect. Dis.* 2010;51:1167-75. Epub 2010 Oct 11.
[64] Weekly update on oseltamivir resistance to pandemic influenza A (H1N1) 2009 viruses. Geneva: World Health Organization, 2010. (http://www.who.int/csr/disease/swineflu/oseltamivirresistant20100611.pdf.).
[65] Emergency use authorization of Peramivir IV: fact sheet for healthcare providers. Atlanta: Centers for Disease Control and Prevention, 2009. (Accessed April 9, 2010, at http://www.cdc.gov/h1n1flu/eua/final%20Fact%20sheet%20Peramivir%20IV_CDC.pdf.).
[66] Kidd IM, Down J, Nastouli E, et al. H1N1 pneumonitis treated with intravenous zanamivir. *Lancet* 2009;374:1036.
[67] Gaur AH, Bagga B, Barman S, et al. Intravenous zanamivir for oseltamivir-resistant 2009 H1N1 influenza. *N. Engl. J. Med.* 2010; 362:88-9.
[68] Update on oseltamivir-resistant pandemic A (H1N1) 2009 influenza virus: January 2010. *Wkly. Epidemiol. Rec.* 2009; 85:37-40.
[69] Noah MA, Peek GJ, Finney SJ, et al. Referral to an extracorporeal membrane oxygenation center and mortality among patients with severe 2009 influenza A(H1N1). *JAMA* 2011;306:1659-68.
[70] Combes A, Pellegrino V. Extracorporeal membrane oxygenation for 2009 influenza A (H1N1)-associated acute respiratory distress syndrome. *Semin. Respir. Crit. Care Med.* 2011;32:188-94.
[71] Nabeshima S, Kashiwagi K, Ajisaka K, et al. A randomized, controlled trial comparing traditional herbal medicine and neuraminidase inhibitors in the treatment of seasonal influenza. *Infect. Chemother.* 2012; 18:534-43. Epub 2012 Feb 16.
[72] Wang C, Cao B, Liu QQ, et al. Oseltamivir compared with the Chinese traditional therapy maxingshigan-yinqiaosan in the treatment of H1N1 influenza: a randomized trial. *Ann. Intern. Med.* 2011;155:217-25.
[73] Mori K, Kido T, Daikuhara H, et al. Anti-viral effect of Hochu-ekki-to (TJ-41), on the model of mice infected with influenza virus. *Journal of Traditional Medicines* 1998;15:370-1. Japanese.

[74] Takagi Y, Higashi N, Maeda A, et al. The effect of crude drug for viral infection-The effect of Mao-bushi-saishin-to on the activity of phagocytic cells in the elderly mouse-. *Kampo to saishin-chiryo* 2001; 1:79-83. Japanese.

[75] Gaur AH, Bagga B, Barman S, et al. Intravenous Zanamivir for Oseltamivir-Resistant 2009 H1N1 Influenza. *N. Engl. J. Med.* 2010; 362: 8-89.

In: Swine Flu ISBN: 978-1-62618-363-6
Editors: J. C. Marie and T. B. Johnson

Chapter 3

SWINE FLU: SIGNS/SYMPTOMS, IMAGING FEATURES AND TREATMENT OPTIONS

***Daphne J. Theodorou*[1,*], *Stavroula J. Theodorou*[2,†], *John Iliodromitis*[1], *Fotios Mantzoukis*[1], *Konstantinos Gossios*[1] *and Nikolaos Akritidis*[3]**

[1]Department of Radiology, General Hospital of Ioannina and National Healthcare System, Ioannina, Greece
[2]Department of Radiology, University Hospital of Ioannina, Ioannina, Greece
[3]Department of Internal Medicine, General Hospital of Ioannina and National Healthcare System, Ioannina, Greece

ABSTRACT

Influenza - A virus of swine origin, H1N1, is a highly contagious virus that has been rapidly transmitted and spread among humans in many countries causing a global pandemic. Clinical manifestations of disease range from asymptomatic infection to mild upper respiratory illness, or severe pneumonia to acute respiratory distress syndrome (ARDS) with progression to multi-organ failure, and an adverse outcome. Populations at increased risk for morbidity and mortality include the very

* Corresponding author: Daphne J. Theodorou, MD, PhD. 13 Papadopoulos street. Ioannina, 45444, Greece. Ph/fax: +302651038003. Email: daphne_theodorou@hotmail.com.

† E-mail: rjtheodorou@hotmail.com.

young and elderly, the pregnant, individuals with comorbid chronic cardiopulmonary conditions, and the immunocompromized. In early stages or in mild cases of infection, chest radiographs can appear normal. With progression of lung infection, typical radiographic and CT findings of the H1N1 viral infection include bilateral, multifocal areas of consolidation associated with ground-glass opacities, in the absence of pleural effusion or lymphadenopathy. Experience from many clinical cases has shown that extensive involvement of both lungs is invariably associated with an adverse prognosis. Recognition of the imaging findings of lung infection (albeit nonspecific for H1N1 viral pneumonia) when associated with clinical and laboratory results may have significance, in the prediction of clinical outcome.

INTRODUCTION

Swine-origin influenza A (H1N1), better known as swine flu, was declared by the World Health Organization as a global pandemic, in June 2009. The highly contagious influenza A H1N1 virus can cause either a mild influenza-like infection that is similar to seasonal influenza, or less frequently, a rapidly progressing community-acquired pneumonic illness that can cause acute respiratory failure and even death. Fortunately, although the virus continues to spread with a high transmission among humans in many countries throughout the world, its virulence by and large is not greater than that observed with seasonal influenza. Large-scale reports of hospitalized patients with H1N1 influenza infection in the United States have addressed severe illness, including respiratory failure and sepsis, in patients with underlying medical conditions, although severe illness was also prevalent among young and previously healthy individuals.

The most common clinical signs and symptoms for H1N1 virus infection are fever, cough, dyspnea, headache, and myalgia. Diagnosing influenza A H1N1 virus pneumonia on chest radiographs and CT scans is important as imaging findings may correlate with severity of the disease and can have relevance in helping predict clinical outcome. Bilateral, symmetric and multifocal areas of consolidation, with or without ground-glass opacities, are the most common—albeit not pathognomonic, radiographic features in patients with the swine flu [1]. Finally, positive findings for influenza A H1N1 virus infection are appreciated on reverse transcriptase polymerase chain reaction or viral culture assays to confirm diagnosis.

Although the imaging findings of pulmonary H1N1 infection are not specific for the diagnosis, association with clinical and laboratory data can be of great value in establishing diagnosis and treating the disease, in any given case. In this chapter, we will provide an integrated review of the clinical presentations of swine influenza, with emphasis on the imaging characteristics of the disease. Furthermore, available treatment options for management of lung infection will be discussed.

ETIOLOGY

Influenza viruses are human pathogens that are responsible for seasonal epidemics and occasional pandemics. Swine-origin influenza, or "swine flu", is a highly contagious acute respiratory disease of pigs that is caused by one of several swine influenza A viruses. Influenza A viruses belong to the family *Orthomyxovirus*, with 16 varieties of hemagglutinin and 9 varieties of neuraminidase proteins used for subtyping. Influenza A pandemics occurred three times in the 20th century: H1N1 in 1918, H2N2 in 1957, and H3N2 in 1968. Of those, the deadliest pandemic in recorded history was that of 1918, with H1N1 viral infection taking a death toll of an estimated 50 million people worldwide, within days of infection [2]. H1N1 re-emerged in 1977 to periodically circulate with H2N2 subtypes as "seasonal flu"[3].

In March 2009, a major outbreak of respiratory disease was reported in Mexico. One month later, a new influenza A virus, H1N1, was detected in California in the United States. This novel H1N1 virus was initially termed "swine origin influenza virus" but further studies revealed that it represented a quadruple reassortment of gene sequences from North American and European human, avian and swine strains [4, 5]. Within few weeks, the virus spread globally, with 254,206 cases having been documented as of September 2009, and an estimated 2,837 deaths [6]. On June 11 2009, the World Health Organization (WHO) declared the H1N1 infection as a global influenza pandemic [7].

Although it remains a significant threat to vulnerable populations, epidemiologic data suggest that the 2009 influenza A (H1N1) virus exhibited relatively low virulence in comparison with the 1918 strain [8]. Reportedly, swine influenza tends to be associated with high morbidity and low mortality (1-4%) [9]. The world is now in the post-pandemic period. On the basis of past pandemics however, the H1N1 (2009) virus is expected to continue to circulate as a seasonal virus for some years to come causing variable levels of disease and outbreaks [10]. WHO strongly recommends vaccination of high-risk individuals in countries where influenza vaccines are available.

Clinical and Laboratory Findings

Epidemiologic data suggest that the H1N1 virus is of relatively low virulence [8] although it may exhibit variable pathogenicity. In some patients even casual exposure can cause symptoms, whereas others appear unaffected even by extensive exposure. Children and young adults are the most susceptible to infection. High-risk groups for complications include pregnant women, adults older than 65 years, children younger than 5 years, and patients with various underlying conditions such as chronic obstructive pulmonary disease (COPD), cardiovascular, renal or chronic liver diseases, hematological disorders, immunosuppression, and metabolic diseases (i.e., diabetes mellitus and obesity) [1, 11]. It is therefore important that clinicians be able to recognize probable cases of H1N1 influenza in high-risk groups so that they order the appropriate diagnostic tests, institute specific antiviral therapy, and provide intensive supportive measures as needed.

Influenza A H1N1 virus can cause either a mild influenza-type infection that is indistinguishable from seasonal influenza, or a rapidly progressive, community-acquired pneumonia [4]. The most common clinical manifestations for H1N1 virus infection at presentation include flu-like symptoms such as fever, chills, cough, sore throat, dyspnea, headache, myalgia, and fatigue [11]. Additional symptoms include nausea, vomiting, and diarrhea. Most cases are mild and self-limited; however, a small percentage of individuals have a severe course that may result in respiratory failure and death. Severe complications may include secondary invasive bacterial infections, septic shock, acute renal failure, reversible cardiac dysfunction, and the multiple organ failure syndrome [1, 4]. A severe course and fatal outcome are more frequent in patients with concomitant chronic diseases as asthma, COPD or congestive heart failure but also can occur in previously healthy individuals.

In terms of laboratory findings, biochemical tests may show elevated lactate dehydrogenase (LDH) levels, increased creatinine-phosphokinase and transaminases levels, lymphopenia or leucopenia or leucocytosis, and thrombocytopenia. The diagnostic test of choice is H1N1 specific, real-time reverse transcriptase polymerase chain reaction (RT-PCR) assay [12-14]. According to the guidelines of the Centers for Disease Control and Prevention

(CDC) samples must be collected through nasopharyngeal aspirate, or nasopharyngeal or pharyngeal swab, or, in the case of pneumonia, through the lower respiratory tract [15, 16].

Histopathologic studies have showed that the acute stage of H1N1 viral infection is characterized by multifocal destruction and desquamation of the tracheal and bronchial epithelia, with marked edema and congestion of the submucosa. There is severe necrotizing bronchiolitis characterized by necrosis of the bronchiolar wall, along with exudative diffuse alveolar damage, interstitial edema and peribronchial hemorrhage, as well as peribronchial pneumonia [17-19]. Severe influenza is characterized by necrotizing bronchitis, capillary thrombosis, alveolar and interstitial edema and inflammatory mononuclear cell infiltrates, the formation of hyaline membranes, and hemorrhage [17-19]. Occasionally, patients may develop thrombosis of the pulmonary arteries. In the latter stages of infection, fibrosing and organizing diffuse alveolar damage may be present. Reportedly, patients with necrotizing bronchiolitis may present a neutrophil-predominant inflammatory exudate indicative of bacterial co-infection [20]. Lung immunopathologic examination has showed marked expression of toll-like receptor (TLR)-3 and IFN-γ and a large number of CD8+ T cells and granzyme B+ cells within the infected lung tissue [17, 20].

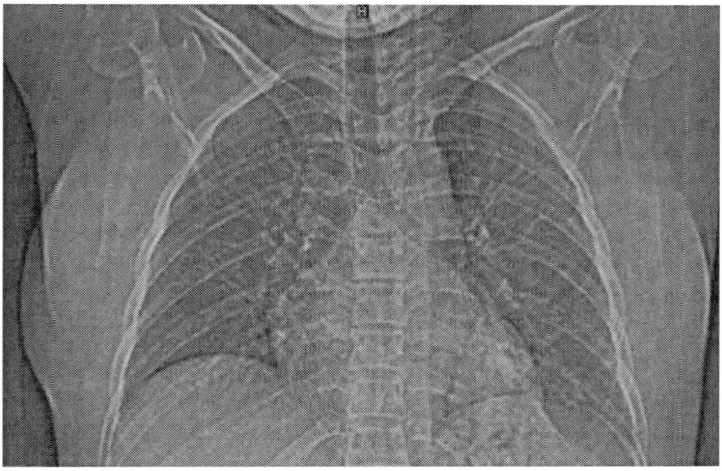

a

Figure 1. (Continued).

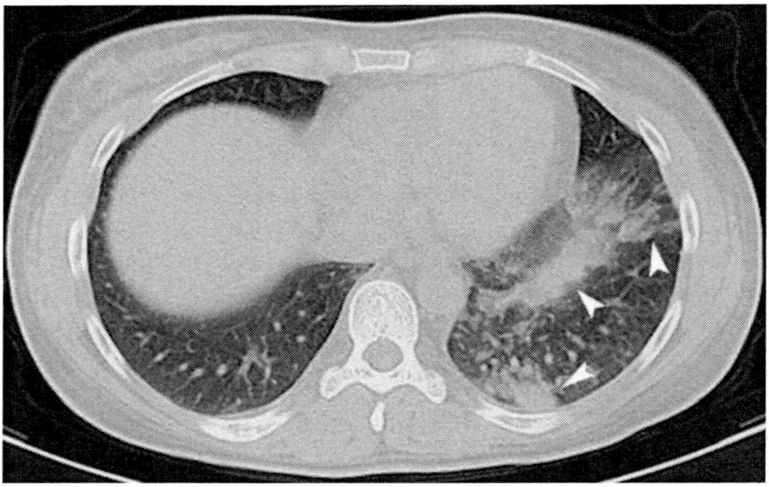

b

Figure 1. 34-year-old woman with mild H1N1 influenza infection presented to emergency department with fever, cough, and arthralgias. A. Chest radiograph shows normal lungs. B. CT image shows confluent consolidations (arrowheads) in left lower lobe, and peripheral ground-glass opacities. Right lung is normal.

IMAGING FINDINGS

Imaging is considered to be fundamental in establishing the diagnosis of pneumonia, and describing its characteristics, extent and distribution. Assessment of the extent of the infectious process in lung may have significance in helping formulate the most appropriate type of treatment and predict clinical outcome. However, normal initial radiographs cannot exclude adverse outcome. In this regard, thin-section computed tomography is used to determine whether lung parenchyma abnormalities are present.

Definitive diagnosis cannot be made on the basis of imaging findings alone, requiring use of a combination of clinical, laboratory and imaging data.

Radiography and Computed Tomography (CT) Findings

i) Parenchymal Changes

In the early stages or mild cases of H1N1 influenza infection, chest radiographs can appear normal (Figure 1). Agarwal et al [21] reported unremarkable chest radiographs in more than half of patients with H1N1 infection. As with viral pneumonias, pneumonia due to influenza virus may appear on serial radiographs as poorly defined, patchy areas of air-space consolidation, which rapidly become confluent [22]. On computed tomography (CT) images, patchy or diffuse areas of ground-glass opacity mixed with consolidation are seen. These multifocal areas of air-space opacities becoming confluent, in essence, reflect combinations of variable histopathologic features including diffuse alveolar damage, hemorrhage, and organizing pneumonia.

Spread of infection and inflammatory exudate in the air-spaces and along the bronchovascular bundles may produce a reticular or reticulonodular pattern [18]. Pleural effusion is usually absent. A superimposed secondary bacterial infection may eventually ensue [18].

CT is more sensitive than radiography in the evaluation of abnormal lung parenchymal findings. The cardinal CT findings in patients with H1N1 infection are ground-glass opacities, areas of consolidation, or a mixed pattern of ground-glass opacities and areas of consolidation [23] (Figures 2, 3). Parenchymal abnormalities are often bilateral and may have a peripheral subpleural, peribronchovascular, lobular, or random distribution (Figure 4). Changes may also be diffuse or, more rarely, unilateral.

Although none of these patterns is specific of H1N1 infection, the main patterns of disease that are most suggestive of H1N1 are scattered lung consolidations, ground-glass opacities, or both, in a peribronchovascular or subpleural distribution, small nodules, and interlobular septal thickening [1, 11, 23] (Figures 5-8).

Scattered or diffuse ground-glass attenuation with superimposed interlobular septal thickening and intralobular lines is termed the "crazy-paving" pattern of involvement on CT of the lungs [4, 23].

ii) Extraparenchymal Changes

Additional extraparenchymal abnormalities have been reported in patients with pulmonary H1N1 infection as well. These include pulmonary embolism, pneumothorax or pneumomediastinum caused by ruptured parenchymal lung cysts associated with severe alveolar damage, and small unilateral or bilateral pleural effusions [21, 23] (Figure 9). Notably, there are no associated lymphadenopathy or pericardial effusions in those patients with H1N1 infection [21].

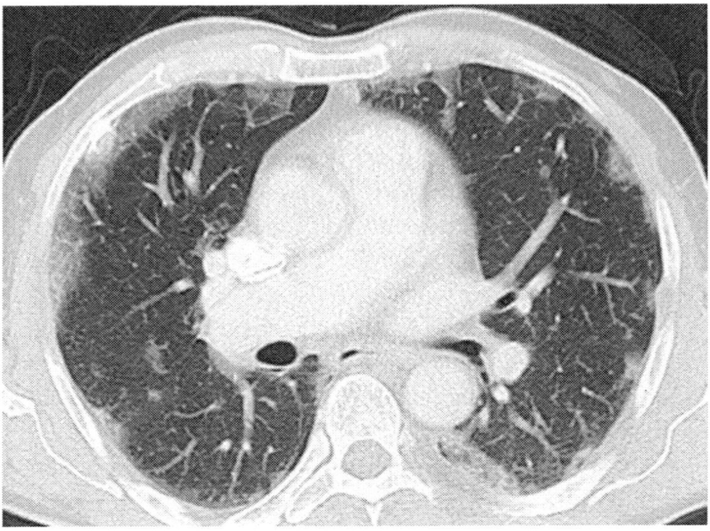

Figure 2. 54-year-old febrile man with H1N1 pneumonia. Axial CT image shows bilateral and predominantly peripheral, focal ground-glass opacities in both lungs.

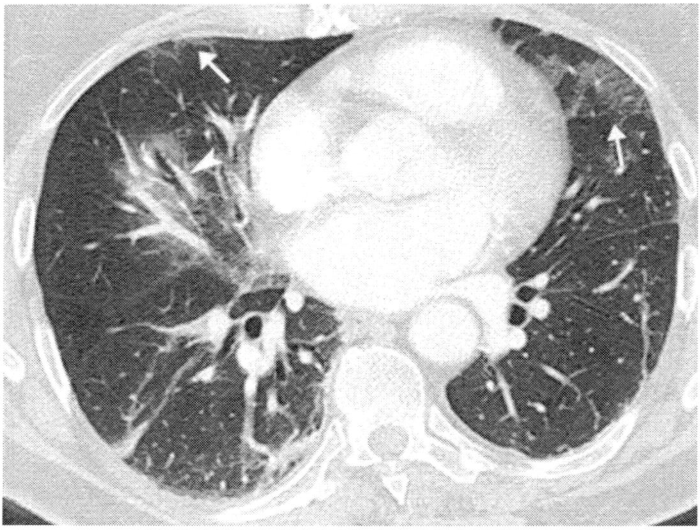

Figure 3. 54-year-old woman with multiple sclerosis and H1N1 pneumonia. Axial CT image of lungs obtained at level of lower lobes shows bilateral, peripheral focal ground -glass opacities in both lungs (arrows). Consolidation with peribronchovascular distribution in right middle lobe is present (arrowhead).

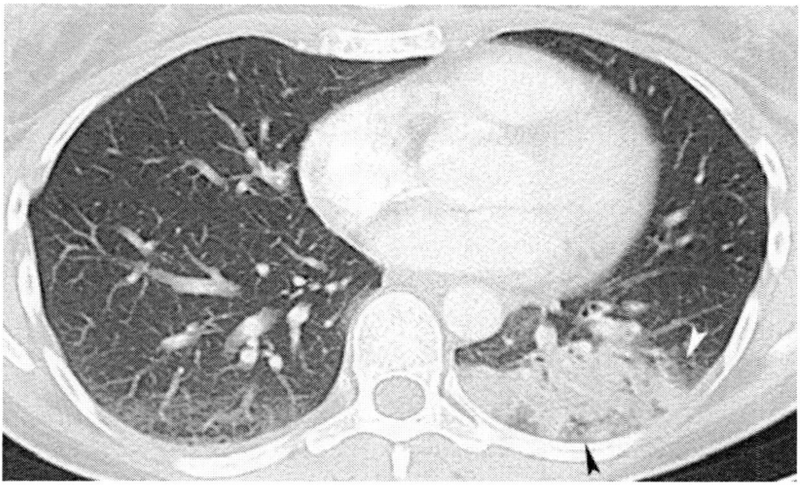

Figure 4. 35-year-old immunocompetent woman with H1N1 pneumonia. Axial CT image shows consolidation with air bronchograms and ground-glass opacity (black arrowhead) in left lower lobe. Note discrete ground-glass halo (halo sign) (white arrowhead).

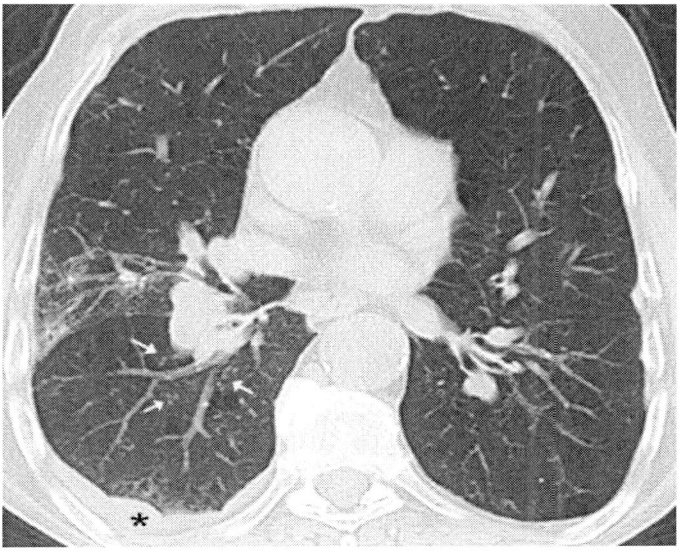

Figure 5. 52-year-old man with lung emphysema and H1N1 pneumonia. Axial CT scan shows ground-glass opacity in a peribronchovascular distribution, in right lung. There are confluent lung nodules (tree-in-bud pattern) (arrows) and a small pleural effusion (asterisk).

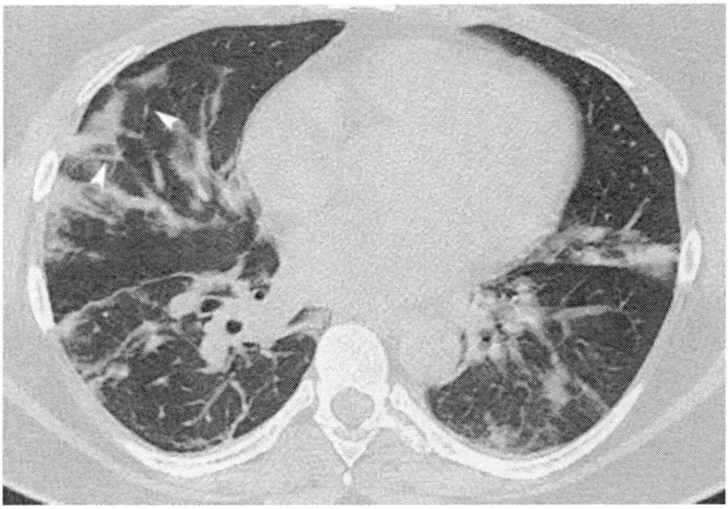

Figure 6. 32-year-old immunocompetent woman with H1N1 pneumonia. Axial CT image of lungs shows peripheral and peribronchovascular consolidations in both lungs, and smooth septal thickening in middle lobe (arrowheads).

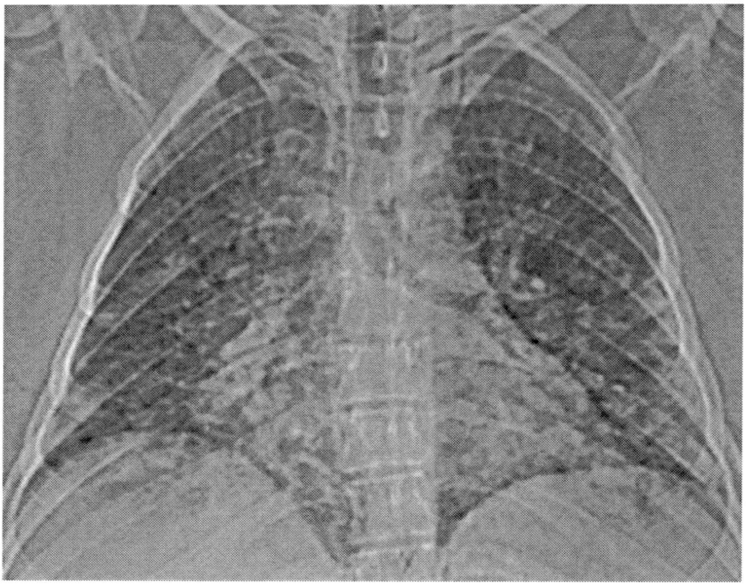

a

Figure 7. (Continued).

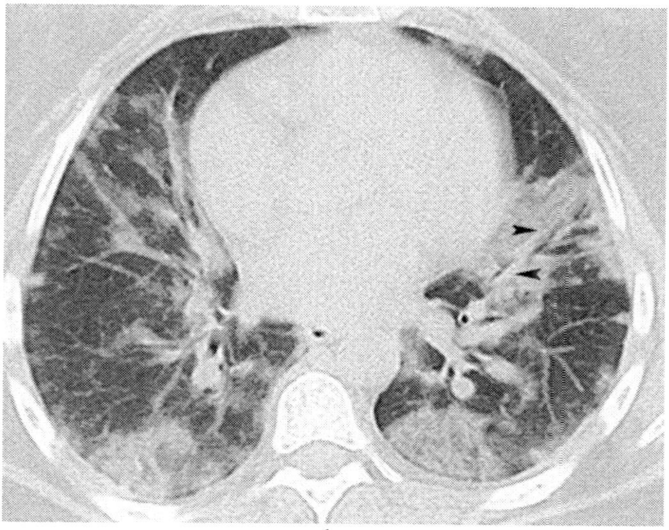

b

Figure 7. 41-year-old immunocompetent woman with H1N1 pneumonia. A. Chest radiograph at clinical presentation shows multifocal opacities, in both lungs. B. Axial CT scan shows bilateral patchy consolidations with air bronchograms (arrowheads) and ground-glass opacities, in subpleural and peribronchovascular distribution.

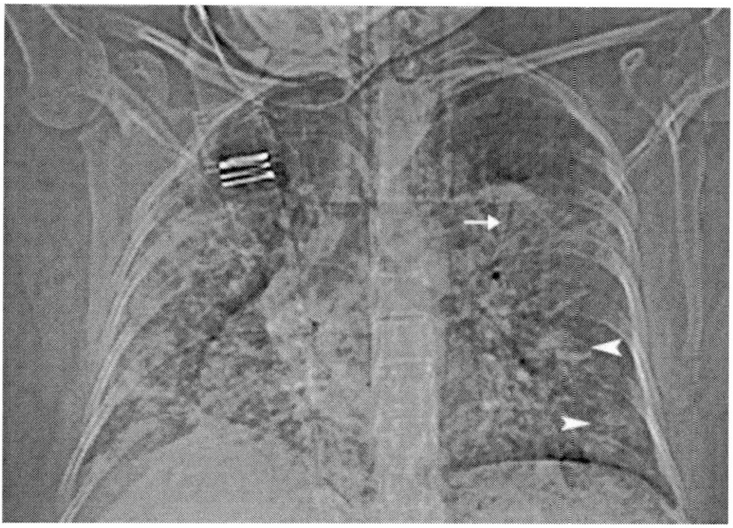

a

Figure 8. (Continued).

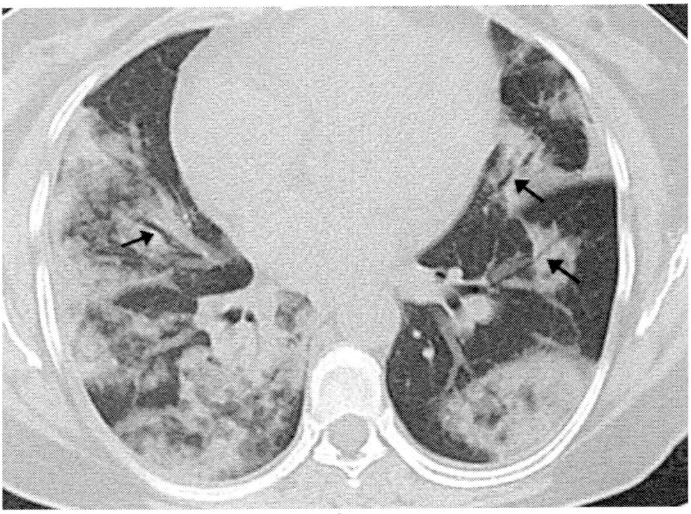

b

Figure 8. 40-year-old woman with H1N1 pneumonia requiring extracorporeal life support. Patient recovered uneventfully. A. Scout image from chest CT examination shows nodular consolidations (arrowheads) and patchy ground-glass opacities. Air-bronchograms are visible on left side (arrow). B. Axial CT scan shows scattered consolidations and nodular opacities in lung parenchyma, with air-bronchograms (arrows).

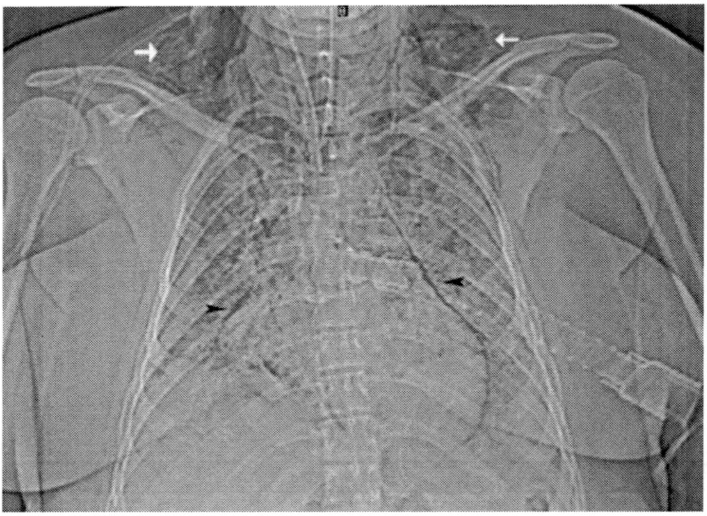

a

Figure 9. (Continued).

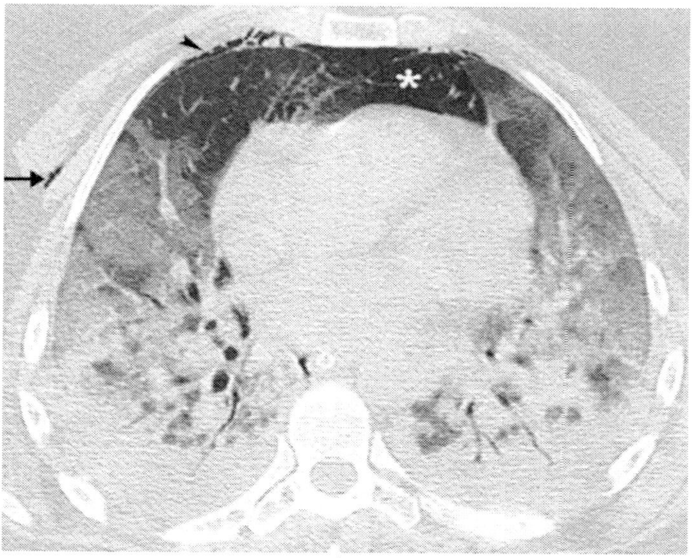

b

Figure 9. 41-year-old woman (same patient as in Figure 7) with H1N1 pneumonia requiring advanced mechanical ventilation with fatal outcome. A. Scout image from chest CT examination obtained 9 days after onset of symptoms shows widespread air-space disease, pneumomediastinum (arrowheads), and subcutaneous emphysema (arrows). B. Axial CT scan (lung window setting) shows bilateral patchy areas of consolidation with air bronchograms and ground-glass opacities. Pneumomediastinum (asterisk), small pneumothorax (arrowhead), and subcutaneous emphysema (arrow) are also seen.

Differential Diagnosis

Imaging findings of peripheral, scattered areas of lung consolidation, ground-glass opacities, or both in a peribronchovascular or subpleural distribution are not specific for H1N1 viral pneumonia. Imaging findings are important, however, when associated with clinical symptoms, contact history, and laboratory data. On the basis of similar imaging appearances, differential diagnosis includes atypical pneumonia (*Mycoplasma, Chlamydia, Legionella*), septic emboli, and other forms of pneumonia as cryptogenic organizing pneumonia (COP), and chronic eosinophilic pneumonia (CEP). Sudden onset of symptoms in H1N1 pneumonia helps differentiate influenza A (H1N1) viral infection from COP and CEP. Furthermore, the clinical differential diagnosis of H1N1 pneumonia may include other viral, bacterial, mycobacterial, and fungal infections. Clinical and laboratory results, and the typical absence of pleural effusion, lymphadenopathy, and lobar consolidation can help eliminate the broad differential diagnosis [24]. Although the imaging findings of H1N1 virus pneumonia usually overlap with those of other infections, the presence of diffuse lung consolidations and ground-glass opacities, in a peribronchovascular or subpleural distribution can be strongly correlated to H1N1 infection [11, 23].

In patients with AIDS, H1N1 infection causing ground-glass opacities may be confused with pneumonia caused by *Pneumocystis jiroveci*, cytomegalovirus pneumonia, lymphocytic interstitial pneumonia, and nonspecific interstitial pneumonia. Similarly, imaging findings are not specific for diagnosis and need to be correlated to clinical and laboratory results for making accurate diagnosis, staging the disease, assessing complications, and following up patients.

Clinical Course

Most influenza A (H1N1) infections in healthy individuals are self-limited. Patients with widespread consolidations have a more severe clinical course than those with less extensive involvement of the lungs [4]. Indeed, it appears that multifocal bilateral opacities and involvement of many lobes in the lung are associated with severe illness and complications that may necessitate mechanical ventilation. Nicolini et al [4] reported that higher serum levels of lactate dehydrogenase (LDH) or lower PaO_2 and PaO_2/FIO_2 ratio correlated directly with severe lung involvement -as observed also on chest CT scans of patients with H1N1 influenza- and use of mechanical ventilation.

In patients with severe H1N1 infection, dyspnea usually progresses rapidly within 24 hours after 5 to 7 days of influenza-like illness, causing severe hypoxemia and ARDS. Bloody respiratory secretions can be present [5]. Lymphopenia, increased serum LDH, creatine kinase, and aminotransferase levels are common laboratory findings in most severe cases [20]. Because patients with progressive symptoms may deteriorate very rapidly (within hours), close observation and rapid intervention in the form of mechanical ventilation or intubation are often required.

Concurrent bacterial infections may develop in severely ill patients with H1N1 influenza. Susceptibility to bacterial co-infection may be due to damage of the defense barrier of the respiratory tract caused by H1N1 virus, or by the inflammatory response. Critically ill patients develop refractory hypoxia and multi-organ system failure, with a fatal outcome [20].

TREATMENT OPTIONS

The World Health Organization (WHO) recommends that healthy individuals with uncomplicated influenza need not treatment with antiviral therapy. However, high-risk patients or severely infected individuals are advised to be treated with neuraminidase inhibitors oseltamivir (Tamiflu; Roche, Switzerland) or zanamivir (Relenza; GlaxoSmithKline, United Kingdom), ideally within 48 hours of the onset of illness [18, 25]. A retrospective cohort study of mild cases of H1N1 infection indicated that with early initiation of therapy (≤2 days after onset of symptoms), oseltamivir could effectively suppress viral load and shorten duration of fever by 1.4 days. When compared to patients whose treatments were initiated more than 2 days after symptom onset, viral shedding was shortened by 1 day in a group that had early treatment with oseltamivir [26]. Older antiviral agents amantadine and rimantadine can block virus surface proteins, but many influenza strains have developed resistance against these medications.

Data from WHO report development of oseltamivir-resistant influenza A (H1N1) viruses, exhibiting an H275Y mutation [27]. The risk of resistance to the antiviral agent is considered higher in patients who have prolonged illness (i.e., immunosuppressed patients), and in those patients who have received antiviral treatment for an extended duration, but still test positive for the virus [25].

Treatment of infection with corticosteroids remains controversial as steroids may produce immunosuppression and increase susceptibility of patients to secondary infections, and may also increase the viral shedding time [18, 25]. Conversely, administration of steroids has been reported to decrease mortality in cases of severe avian (H5N1) influenza and severe acute respiratory syndrome (SARS) by reducing an exuberant systemic inflammatory response incited by these viruses [28].

In severely ill patients with respiratory failure where oxygen saturation cannot be maintained over 90% by mechanical ventilation, extracorporeal membrane oxygenation may need to be used [29].

Conclusion

As with viral pneumonias in general, pulmonary H1N1 infection can present with variable radiographic and CT imaging patterns, none of which is specific for the diagnosis. Patchy or diffuse ground-glass opacity, with or without consolidation, in a peripheral or peribronchovascular distribution are among the features most characteristic of the infection. Patient age, immune status, community outbreaks, clinical symptoms onset and duration, and laboratory test results are important in diagnosis of H1N1 infection.

References

[1] Theodorou D. J., Theodorou S. J., Tsoumani A., Gossios K. Akritidis N. Radiographic and CT findings in pandemic swine-origin influenza A (H1N1). *Europ J Internal Med* 2010;21:e7–e8.

[2] Taubenberger J., Morens D. 1918 influenza: the mother of all pandemics. *Emerg Infect Dis* 2006;12 (1):15–22.

[3] Peiris J., Poon L., Guan Y. Emergence of a novel swine-origin influenza A virus (S-OIV) virus in humans. *J Clin Virol* 2009;45:169-173.

[4] Nicolini A., Ferrera L., Rao F., Senarega R., Ferrari-Bravo M. Chest radiological findings of influenza A H1N1 pneumonia. *Rev Port Pneumol* 2012;18(3):120-127.

[5] Perez-Padilla R., de la Rosa-Zamboni D., Ponce de Leon S., Hernandez M., Quinones-Falconi F., Bautista E. etal. Pneumonia and respiratory failure from swine-origin influenza A (H1N1) in Mexico. *N Engl J Med* 2009;361:680-689.

[6] World Health Organization Website. *Global alert and response: Pandemic (H1N1) 2009*: Update 64. www.who.int/csr/don/2009-09-04/en/index.html.

[7] World Health Organization WHO. *World now at start of 2009 influenza pandemic*. www.who.int/mediacentre/news/statements/2009/h1n1_pandemic_phase 6_20090611/en/index.html.

[8] Centers for Disease Control and Prevention (CDC). Update: novel influenza A (H1N1) virus infections-worldwide, May 6, 2009. *MMWR Morb Mortal Wkly Rep* 2009; 58:453-458.

[9] World Health Organization Website. *Weekly epidemiological record*: 2009; 84, No 18:149-160 www.who.int/csr/disease/swineflu/en/index.html.

[10] World Health Organization Website. Global alert and response (GAR). *WHO recommendations for the post-pandemic period*. Briefing note 23. www.who.int/csr/disease/swineflu/notes/briefing-20100810/en/index.html.

[11] Ajlan A., Quiney B., Nicolaou S., Muller N. Swine-origin influenza A (H1N1) viral infection: Radiographic and CT findings. *Am J Roentgenol* 2009;193:1494-1499.

[12] Franquet T. Imaging of pulmonary viral pneumonia. *Radiology* 2011; 260:18-39.

[13] Carr M., Gunson R., Maclean A., et al. Development of a real-time RT-PCR for the detection of swine-lineage influenza A (H1N1) virus infections. *J Clin Virol* 2009;45(3):196-199.

[14] Whiley D., Bialasiewicz S., Bletchly C. et al. Detection of novel influenza A (H1N1) virus by real-time RT-PCR. *J Clin Virol* 2009; 45 (3):203-204.

[15] U. S. Centers for Disease Control and Prevention Website. *Interim guidance on specimen collection, processing and testing for patients with suspected novel influenza A (H1N1) virus infection.* www.cdc.gov/h1n1flu/specimencollection.htm. Published May 13, 2009.

[16] World Health Organization Website. *Global alert and response: CDC protocol of realtime RTPCR for influenza A* (H1N1). www.who.int/csr/resources/publications/swineflu/realtimeptpcr/en/index.html. Published April 30, 2009.

[17] Mauad T., Hajjar L., Callegari G. et al. Lung pathology in fatal novel human influenza A (HN1) infection. *Am J Respir Crit Care Med* 2010; 181:72-79.

[18] Guo H., Sweeney R., Regula D., Leung A. Fatal 2009 influenza A (H1N1) infection, complicated by acute respiratory distress syndrome and pulmonary interstitial emphysema. *Radiographics* 2010;30:327-333.

[19] Taubenberger J., Morens D. The pathology of influenza virus infections. *Annu Rev Pathol* 2008;3:499-522.

[20] Bai L., Cao B., Wanf C. Influenza A pandemic (H1N1) 2009 virus infection. *Chinese Medical Journal* 2011;124(20):3399-3402.

[21] Agarwal P., Cinti S., Kazerooni E. Chest radiographic and CT findings in novel swine-origin influenza A (H1N1) virus (S-OIV) infection. *Am J Roentgenol* 2009;193:1488-1493.

[22] Kim E., Lee K., Primack S., Yoon H., Byun H., Kim T., Suh G., Kwon O., Han J. Viral pneumonias in adults: Radiologic and pathologic findings. *Radiographics* 2002;22:S137-S149.

[23] Marchiori E., Zanetti G., D'Ippolito G., Verrastro C., Meirelles G., Capobianco J., Rodrigues R. Swine-origin influenza A (H1N1) viral infection: Thoracic findings on CT. *Am J Roentgenol* 2011;196:723-728.

[24] Aviram G., Ba-Shai A., Sosna J., Rogowski O., Rosen G., Weinstein J., Steinvil A., Zimmerman O. H1N1 influenza: Initial chest radiographic findings in helping predict patient outcome. *Radiology* 2010;255;252-259.

[25] World Health Organization WHO. *Clinical management of human infection with pandemic (H1N1)* 2009: Revised guidance. www.who.int/csr/resources/publications/swineflu/clinical-management-1n1. pdf.

[26] Li I., Hung I., To K., Chan K., Wong S., Chan J. et al. The natural viral load profile of patients with pandemic 2009 influenza A (H1N1) and the effect of oseltamivir treatment. *Chest* 2010;137:759-768.

[27] World Health Organization WHO. Pandemic (H1N1) 2009. update 91. *Virological surveillance data*. www.who.int/csr/disease/swineflu/ laboratory 12-03-2010/en/index.html.

[28] Chen R., Tang X., Tan S. et al. Treatment of severe acute respiratory syndrome with glucosteroids: the Guangzhou experience. *Chest* 2006; 129(6):1441-1452.

[29] Davies A., Jones D., Bailey M., Beca J., Bellomo R., Blackwell N. et al. Extracorporeal membrane oxygenation for 2009 influenza A (H1N1) acute respiratory distress syndrome. *JAMA* 2009;302:1888-1895.

In: Swine Flu
Editors: J. C. Marie and T. B. Johnson
ISBN: 978-1-62618-363-6

Chapter 4

TREATMENT AND MONITORING OF THE SEVERE INFLUENZA A H1N1 INFECTED PATIENTS

Wei Zhao, Xuan Liu and Yishan Zheng
The second affiliated hospital of the South East University, Nanjing, China

ABSTRACT

During the outburst of Influenza A H1N1 in China in 2009, our hospital admitted 232 confirmed cases of Influenza A H1N1, including 67 cases of severely ill patients. All of the 67 severe Influenza A H1N1 cases combined with pneumonia, with 6 cases of unilateral pneumonia and 61 cases of double pneumonia. This section enumerated five typical severely ill cases of Influenza A H1N1, including the combination of respiratory failure and fungal infections, hemophagocytic syndrome, invasive pulmonary aspergillosis, pericardial effusion, and pregnancy. All of the 67 cases of severe Influenza A H1N1 have been successfully cured, except one case of pregnant woman. Herein, the curing methods for the 5 typical severe cases were discussed, with the summarized treatment experiences. The early treatment was with the great importance for the curing of severely ill patients of Influenza A H1N1, and efficient monitoring and treatment could prevent the mild Influenza A H1N1 developing to severe conditions. Ventilator supporting and glucocorticoids treatment could be used for curing of Influenza A H1N1infection at specific indicators.

Keywords: Influenza A H1N1; treatment and monitoring; severe

INTRODUCTION

In September 2009, the H1N1 virus had already spread in many countries around the world [1,2]. Influenza A H1N1 virus is influenza virus, which spread mainly by the droplets through the respiratory tract, also transmitted through direct or indirect contact via the mucosa of oral cavity, nasal cavity, eyes and so on. The Influenza A H1N1 virus is considered as the main source of infection. The population is generally susceptible to this virus. The high-risk groups were prone to have severe tendency, leading to respiratory failure, multiple organs failure, pneumonia and other complications after infection. In some cases, the original underlying disease could be aggravated by the Influenza A H1N1 infection, showing the corresponding clinical manifestations.

Usually, for the Influenza A H1N1 infected patients, the mortality rate is about 0.4%, while for the severely ill patients with various complications, the mortality rate showed a large increasing. Most of these patients were young, pregnant, and had various conditions including asthma, diabetes, and heart, lung or neurologic disease (pneumonia ~40%) [3]. Clinical data have also shown that the obesity is another key risk factor [4]. To the patients with persisting viral infections, secondary bacterial infections may occur with the risk of secondary pneumonia, which should be treated by antibiotics [5].

In general, there is a tendency to develop to severe conditions if the Influenza A H1N1 infected population showed flu-like symptoms. In that case, the patients should be given a high attention, and the necessary detections such as H1N1 influenza virus nucleic acid detection should be carried out as soon as possible. The population with the following conditions could be considered as the more susceptible populations:

(1) The pregnant women;
(2) With the following conditions: chronic respiratory disease, cardiovascular disease (except hypertension), kidney disease, liver disease, blood system diseases, nervous system and neuromuscular diseases, metabolic and endocrine system disorders, immune function

suppression (including using immunosuppressive agents cr HIV infection caused by immunocompromised) and the long-term aspirin users less than 19 years old;

(3) Obesity (BMI $\geq$ 40 could be considered with a high risk factcr; BMI between 30 and 39 could be considered with a suspect high risk factor);
(4) The children under 5 years old (especially under 2 years old);
(5) Old people older than 65 years old.

The general situation of Influenza A H1N1 treatments in our hospital and the treatments of typical cases

2.1. The General Situation

During the outbreak of Influenza A H1N1 in 2009 (from June 16 to December 18), there were 232 cases of the Influenza A H1N1 infected patients admitted and treated in our hospital, which was specified as the municipal designated hospital for Influenza A H1N1 treatment. Of these cases, 67 severely ill patients complicated with pneumonia, with 6 cases of unilateral pneumonia and 61 cases of double pneumonia. Among these 67 patients, there were 8 critically ill cases, the complications of whom were listed in Table 1, and the main treatments were listed in Table 2. Most of the inpatients obtained good treatments. The general information and the cure experiences, especially for the 5 typical severely ill cases, were presented in the following contents.

Tabel 1. The complications and their cases of the 8 critically ill patients

Complications	Cases
Gastrointestinal hemorrhage	1
Double pneumonia	8
Respiratory failure	8
Fungal infections	8
Bacterial pneumonia	8
Shock	3
Pneumothorax	4
Hydropericardium	1
Pulmonary hemoptysis	1
Hear failure	2

Tabel 2. The main treatments and their corresponding case and effect for the 67 severely ill patients

Main treatments	Cases	Ratio
Antiviral therapy (Tamiflu)	67	100%
Antibiotic therapy	67	100%
Hormone therapy	6	9%
Noninvasive ventilation	28	42%
Mechanical ventilation	8	12%

2.2. The Treatments of the Typical Cases

Case 1. Influenza A H1N1 Complicated with Respiratory Failure, Fungal Infection and Pulmonary Hemoptysis

Male, fever and cough for one week. The patient had a chill with no obvious incentive on Oct. 1, showing a fever heat peak of 40.4 °C and complicating with a cough. On Oct. 3, the patient received treatment in another hospital at first, and at that time the chest CT investigation showed no abnormal situations. The patient received an anti-infection treatment, while the body temperature did not return to the normal level, and gradually deteriorate to occurring chest tightness, wheezing and bloody sputum. On Oct. 6, the patient had a recurrence of severe asthma and cough. The reexamination of CT showed a lung divergent oozing shadow. The RT of blood showed that WBC was of 8.21×10^9 and neutrophils were of 91.4%. The blood gas analysis showed results with PO of 250 mmhg and PCO_2 of 32.4 mmhg. The patient was given a treatment with methylprednisolone and Tazocin, and the throat swab test of influenza A H1N1 virus nucleic acid was also performed on the same day. On Oct. 7, the patient suffered from significantly worse chest tightness, with conditions of unconsciousness and cyanosis. At the meantime the throat swab H1N1 influenza virus nucleic acid detection obtained a positive result.

Then the patient was transferred to our hospital. Two weeks later, the patient started fever and cough again, with body temperature of 38-39 °C. The sputum smear and sputum fungal culture are Aspergillus flavus possitive, and the drug sensitive test showed sensitivity to caspofungin and voriconazole. The sputum culture showed positive to Escherichia coli (ESBL), which was sensitive to imipenem and Mepem. The chest CT showed multiple empties.

According to the result of drug sensitive test, the patient was given a treatment with tienam and caspofungin, and the symptoms were alleviated.

In the evening of Oct. 30, the patient suddenly had a hemoptysis, with a volume of about 300 mL. The emergency tracheotomy and ventilator supporting were performed and additional 500 mL blood was sucked out from the posterior pituitary via the endotracheal intubation. After that the patient was transferred to the ICU of another hospital in Nanjing and given caspofungin and voriconazole to antifungal treatment. Finally, the patient was recovered.

Case 2. Severe Influenza A H1N1 Complicated with Hemophagocytic Syndrome

Female, 17 years old. The patient was having fever, weakness and coughing for 10 days and was hospitalized on Oct. 10.

Physical examination: The body temperature was of 38.8 °C, with pulse of 135 times/min, respiratory of 44 times/min, blood pulse of 96/51 mmHg and SpO_2 of 64%. The patient showed the appearance of anemia and systemic cyanosis, and the coarse breath sounds and moist rales could be heard in both lungs.

Laboratory tests: Blood count showed results of WBC of 0.6×10^9/L, Hb of 57 g/L and PLT of 31×10^9/L; blood biochemistry test showed a result that TB, ALB, ALT, AST, CK and LDH were of 23 μmol/L, 30 g/L, 23 U/L, 52 U/L, 226 U/L and 3313 U/L, respectively. Fortunately, the electrolytes and renal function were with the normal range. The CT test showed bilateral pulmonary inflammation. After antiviral treatment, ventilation supporting, immune supporting and nutritional support, the double lungs gradually returned to normal and the patient was transferred to another hospital for blood diseases.

Case 3. Influenza A H1N1 Complicated with Aspergillus Infection

Male, 30 years old. The patient was hospitalized on Oct. 30 after keep fevering and coughing up phlegm for 6 days. There was a positive response of throat swabs H1N1 influenza virus nucleic acid detection. After admission, the patient showed a body temperature of 39 °C, with pulse of 105 times/min and SPO_2 of 85%. After non-invasive ventilator supporting, the SPO_2 was maintained at 95%. The twice sputum cultures both showed positive response of Aspergillus, indicating that the patient was complicated with the infection of Aspergillus in double lungs. By the anti-viral, anti-fungal and non-invasive ventilator supporting, the double lungs of the patient returned to normal and the patient was discharged.

Case 4. Influenza A H1N1 Complicated with Pericardial Effusion

Male, 13 years old. The patient was having a high fever, cough and chest tightness for five days, and then was admitted in our hospital. The chest radiograph showed bilateral pulmonary inflammation and a large amount of pericardial effusion. Then the patient was given Tamiflu and Rocephin for anti-viral and anti-infective treatments, respectively. After one week of treatment, the pulmonary symptoms significantly reduced, and the inflammation was obviously absorbed. In addition, the throat swab Influenza A H1N1 virus detection was turned to negative. Then the patient was transferred to another hospital in Nanjing for further treatment of pericardial effusion.

Case 5. Influenza A H1N1 Virus Infected Pregnant Women

The pregnant woman with gestational age of 34 weeks was admitted in our hospital for the gall cholestasis in the liver. The patient complicated with cough and a small amount of white sputum, with the body temperature of 39.4 ^{o}C. The throat swabs influenza A H1N1 virus monitoring showed a positive response. Then the emergency cesarean section was performed and the patient successfully delivered a baby boy. On the next day, the patient got an increase degree of cough and sputum, and the moist rales could be heart in double lungs. The SPO_2 was of 82-83% and the HR was of 120 times/min. The chest X-ray examination showed inflammation on double lungs.

Treatment: Tamiflu was used for antiviral treatment. Imipenem, vancomycin and caspofungin were used for anti-infected treatment. The gamma globulin Zadaxin was used to inhibit the inflammatory response via immune regulation. However, after these treatments the condition of the patient was not improved. On the other hand, there was a severe tendency, with the oxygen saturation showing a progressive decrease. Noninvasive ventilator supporting did not work well, while some deteriorative situations occurred, such as the pneumothorax, acid-base unbalance, electrolyte imbalance, pulmonary hypertension and pulmonary edema. The mediastinotomy was performed for decompression, together with the multiple organs supporting therapy. The conditions of the lung gradually improved, and the parameters of ventilator were gradually decreased. The ventilator was revoked 5 days later, and the bilateral lung inflammation subsided another 5 days later after the endotracheal tube was unpluged. Then the patient recovered and was discharged from the hospital, with a healthy baby. A 3 months following-up indicated that the patient got no complications after discharging.

Compared to the dead pregnant woman (with the gestational age of 18 weeks) infected by the Influenza A H1N1 in our hospital, the successfully curing of this case could be attributed to the emergency cesarean section, and we consider that the intrauterine fetal death might be the key point for death of the Influenza A H1N1 infected pregnant woman.

CONCLUSION

3.1. The Clinic Diagnosis of Severely and Critically Ill Influenza A H1N1 Infection

The patients with one of the following conditions could be diagnosed as severely ill cases:

1. Keep hyperpyrexia for more than 3 days;
2. Serious coughing, coughing purulent sputum or bloody sputum, or chest pain;
3. With rapid respiratory rate, dyspnea and cyanosis of lips;
4. Mental status changing: unresponsive, drowsiness, restlessness, convulsions and so on;
5. Severe vomiting, diarrhea and dehydration;
6. Imaging examinations showed signs of pneumonia;
7. The levels of creatine kinase (CK) and creatine kinase isoenzyme (CK-MB) both increased rapidly;
8. The original underlying diseases aggravated.

The patients with one of the following conditions could be diagnosed as critically ill cases:

1. Respiratory failure;
2. Septic shock;
3. Multiple organs dysfunction;
4. Other serious clinical conditions in need of care.

3.2. The Chest Radiography

The X-ray chest radiographes of general influenza A H1N1 infected patients are always normal. The influenza A H1N1 viral induced severe pneumonia showed a correspondence of increased lung markings and thickening in X-ray chest examination or CT chest scan in the inferior lobe (or double lungs) and the mid-region. Sometimes spotted shadow could be observed, indicating an exudative lesions change; when the lesions near the pleura, the reactive pleural swollen thick showed up, even with a small amount of pleural effusion. The severe influenza A H1N1 could develop to viral pneumonia, sometimes complicated with bacterial pneumonia. In that case, besides the manifestations mentioned above, there could be one or multiple lung segment consolidations on one or multiple lobes. In severely ill cases, acute respiratory distress syndrome (ARDS) would further occur.

3.3. Treatment Principle

1. General Treatment

The patients should rest as much as possible and drink plenty of water. The medical stuff should closely observe the conditions of the patients and give antipyretic treatment of the cases having a high fever.

2. Antiviral Treatment

For the mild cases of Influenza A H1N1 infection without complications, and with the conditions tend to be self-limiting, the patients were unnecessarliy given neuraminidase inhibitors for treatment.

The cases with serious conditions at the onset and showing a dynamic deterioration afterwards could be defined as high-risk groups of the Influenza A H1N1 infection. In that case, the neuraminidase inhibitor should be provided timely for antiviral therapy. Start time of administration should, as far as possible, within 48 hours of the onset (within 36 hours is the best). For the high-risk groups easier to become severe cases, once showing flu-like symptoms, the antiviral therapy should be started immediately, without waiting for the results of viral nucleic acid detection. In addition, once the pregnant women showed the flu-like symptoms, it is advisable to give the neuraminidase inhibitor therapy as early as possible.

The Influenza A H1N1 virus was sensitive to neuraminidase inhibitors, such as oselta mivir and zanamivir, while resistant to amantadine and rimantadine.

3.4 Experiences for the Prevention and Treatment of the Severely Ill Influenza A H1N1 Infection

1. Vigilance and Early Intervention

The conditions of Influenza A H1N1 infected patients usually become severe at the third to fifth day during the disease cause. Thus, if the patients have a fever over 3 days, and the temperature showed no decrease tendency, the chest radiography should be checked timely. The total number of the T lymphocytes and CD4+, CD8+ cells showed a significantly decreasing, resulting in a tendency of co-infection for the patients.

If the patients showed aggravating cough, expectoration and asthma, the chest radiography should be checked and the finger pulse oxygen should be monitored. All of the diagnosed severe cases should take the regular tests of sputum smear, sputum culture, fungal culture and blood culture.

The high-risk factors, such as pregnancy and co-infection should be removed as much as possible.

2. Ventilator Supporting

CT examination should be performed timely. If the characteristic lesions could be observed, the noninvasive respiratory supporting should be given as soon as possible. For the cases that finger pulse oxygen still lower than 90% after the using of oxygen mask, the patients should be supported with noninvasive ventilator, even with the invasive ventilator of the endotracheal intubation when necessary. The positive end-expiratory pressure (PEEP) could mitigate the pulmonary edema and avoid alveolar collapse. The EPAP limited parameter of noninvasive ventilator was usually set no more than 16. Prone position for 45 minutes-146 hours was benefit to alveolar reexpansion of the bottom and back of pulmonary, also to the sputum drainage.

3. Rational Use of Glucocorticoids

The use of glucocorticoids could help to inhibit the allergic reactions and reduce the exudation of pulmonary inflammatory. The early use of glucocorticoids could control the progression of the disease rapidly.

The application indications of glucocorticoids were listed as following:

Complicating septic shock; complicating ARDS, and with hypoxia hard to recover; still having a high fever when the disease cause is longer than 5 days; the radiography or other imaging data showing a lung inflammation stove still in progress.

Dose and course of the treatment should depend on the conditions of the patients: 1-5 mg/kg of Methylprednisolone could be used with sufficient quantities for 3-4 days. After that, if the lung lesions did not progress or showed dissipation, the dose of the Methylprednisolone could be reduced, and the total course should be no more than one week.

When there was a possibility to occur pulmonary fibrosis, the use of hormone could improve lung oxygen exchange.

4. Maintenance of the Aqueous Electrolyte

Once considering the existence of complication of bacteria and fungal infections, it is necessary to provide appropriate treatment for the patients in a timely manner, which could gain more time for the following treatment. It is of the great significance of the maintenance of water and electrolyte balance. The hourly intake and output amount should be accurately calculated, with the measuring of central venous pressure and continuous arterial pressure. Ensure that injecting a certain amount of plasma and protein sufficiently for daily use. The diuretics are appropriate to be injected by a micro pump for 24-hour through the vena. The parenteral nutrition (Calvin) and enteral nutrition (Fresubin) should be supplied timely. The immune modulating drugs such as ntravenous gamma globulin and Zadaxin could be used as appropriate.

In summery, the reasonable application of the critical care supporting technology is a strong guarantee for the cure of the severely and critically ill Influenza A H1N1 infected patients. When it is necessary, the hormones should be used to suppress the inflammation and improve pulmonary symptoms and hypoxemia; strengthen fluid management is important, especially to reduce the lung water load as early as possible; to control the secondary pulmonary infection timely and effectively; to strengthen immune supportive treatment and perform the antiviral treatment as early as possible.

REFERENCES

[1] Franco-Paredes C, Hernandez-Ramos I, Del Rio C, Alexander KT, Tapia-Conyer R, Santos-Preciado JI. H1N1 influenza pandemics:

Comparing the events of 2009 in Mexico with those of 1976 and 1918–1919. *Arch. Med. Res.* 2009, *40*, 669–672.

[2] Economic Review. 2010. Swine flu: facts, symptoms, Diagnosis, prevention, treatment and vaccine. (Disease/Disorder overview) *Economic and Industrial Publications*. High Beam Research (http://www.highbeam.com)

[3] Faruqui F, MukundanD. 2009 Pandemic influenza: *Areview. Curr. Opin. Pediatr.* 2010, *22*, 530-5535.

[4] Gill JR, Sheng ZM, Ely SF, Guinee DG, Beasley MB, Suh J, Deshpande C, Mollura DJ, Morens DM, Bray M, Travis WD, Taubenberger JK. Pulmonary pathologic findings of fatal 2009 pandemic influenza A/H1N1 viral infections. *Arch. Pathol. Lab. Med.* 2010, *134*, 235-243.

[5] Morens DM, Taubenberger JK, Fauci AS. Predominant role of bacterial pneumonia as a cause of death in pandemic influenza: Implications for pandemic influenza preparedness. *J. Infect. Dis.* 2008, *198*, 962-970.

In: Swine Flu
Editors: J. C. Marie and T. B. Johnson
ISBN: 978-1-62618-363-6

Chapter 5

DAVID AGAINST GOLIATH – SOME PUNY RHINOVIRUSES DELAYED THE 2009 INFLUENZA A (H1N1)PDM09 PANDEMIC IN NORWAY?

Gabriel Ånestad*

Department of Virology, Division of Infectious Disease Control,
Norwegian Institute of Public Health, Nydalen, Oslo, Norway

ABSTRACT

During summer and autumn of 2009 Norway, like several other European countries, experienced an unexpected delay in the emergence and spread of the new pandemic influenza A (H1N1)pdm09. It is considered whether interference of other respiratory viruses, in particular rhinoviruses, may have hampered the development of the pandemic, and if interference phenomena are common in the development of outbreaks with epidemic viruses. If so, cytokines, in particular interferon, are the most probable executor of this effect. The virus interference theory may form a reasonable explanation why pandemic influenza, in contrast to seasonal influenza, tends to occur in waves.

* Department of Virology, Division of Infectious Disease Control, Norwegian Institute of Public Health. P.O. Box 4404, Nydalen, N-0403 Oslo, Norway. Tel.: +47 21076284; fax: +47 21076447. E-mail address: gabriel.anestad@fhi.no.

Influenza Virus

A novel strain of influenza A (H1N1) virus, now known as influenza A (H1N1)pdm09 virus, was first identified in Mexico and the United States in April 2009. A rapid spread across the world was observed, and on June 11 WHO declared the first pandemic influenza outbreak in the 21th century.

In Norway the first cases of the influenza A (H1N1)pdm09 virus were detected in the middle of May. During the following weeks an increase was observed in the number of laboratory confirmed cases with the new virus and with only occasional infections with other influenza A (H3N2) and influenza B viruses [1].

In Figure 1, the weekly number of laboratory confirmed cases of influenza are presented together with the proportion of cases with influenza-like illness (ILI). Figure 1 shows that during the 12-week period, from week 30 to 42 (mid July – mid October), there was an unexpected drop in influenza cases, this despite that percent of ILI cases continued to increase until week 35 (late August). From week 43 a sharp increase in influenza virus detections and ILI cases were observed with culmination in week 45.

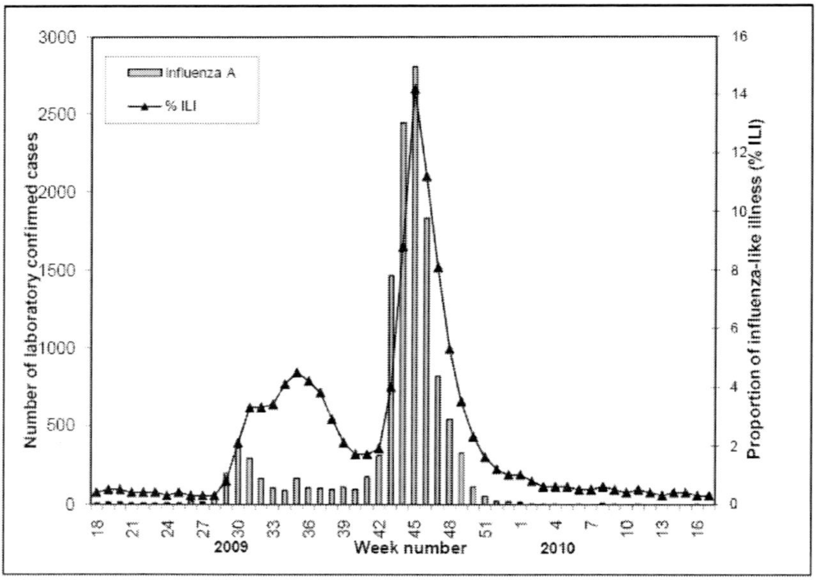

Figure 1. Number of laboratory confirmed cases of influenza A virus, week 18, 2009 – week 17, 2010 in Norway, compared with percent of cases with influenza-like illness (ILI).

Rhinovirus Interference

Sweden experienced a similar delay in the emergence and spread of the influenza A (H1N1)pdm09 virus. A. Linde and co-workers hypothesized that some other virus infections may have interfered with the spread of the influenza A (H1N1)pdm09 virus. They contacted laboratories in Sweden which conducted extended viral diagnosis on samples sent for influenza examination and asked what viruses they found in influenza-negative samples, and the answer was unanimous: rhinoviruses dominated, with sporadic findings of other respiratory viruses, such as enteroviruses and adenoviruses [2].

St. Olavs University Hospital in Trondheim is the main hospital for Mid-Norway. This hospital has for several years conducted extensive virological examinations for respiratory viruses including rhinoviruses. During the summer 2009, a relatively sharp increase in rhinovirus infections was observed from the middle of July. This rhinovirus outbreak was succeeded by influenza and respiratory syncytial virus (RSV) outbreaks with separate peaks [3, 4].

In Lyon, France an early start of rhinovirus outbreaks were observed during the 2008-09 and the 2009-10 winter seasons. In both seasons, the rhinovirus outbreaks were followed by distinct outbreaks of RSV and influenza virus. In 2008-09 came the RSV outbreak before influenza. In the last season, which was dominated by influenza A (H1N1)pdm09, the influenza outbreak before RSV [5] began.

Virus

Like many other respiratory viruses the influenza virus is enveloped with an outer lipid membrane that surrounds the virus capsid. Such viruses are fragile and will be easily damaged if external conditions are unfavorable. Studies have shown that the lipid membrane is most stable in dry and cool weather [6]. This may, at least partly, explain why influenza and other respiratory viruses such as RSV and parainfluenza viruses usually have their main activity during the winter months. Compared with the influenza virus, the rhinovirus has a simple structure with an outer capsid that encloses the nucleic acid. Under unfavorable weather conditions, rhinoviruses have clear advantages over influenza and other complex-built respiratory viruses [3].

If the interference theory is correct, the rhinoviruses may have found their epidemiological niche in late summer and autumn, and thus be able to live in peace and harmony without any competing viruses. So what happens if a new virus suddenly appears that has not found its place in the hierarchy and occurs across these season phases? Then the interference forces are likely to be turned on and result in a delayed epidemiological development of the intruder [3]. In this context, a study by Greer and colleagues [7] must be mentioned. They observed that co-infections with rhinoviruses and other respiratory viruses were less common than expected, indicating that the rhinovirus infection may leave the host less likely to be infected with other viruses.

Is it reasonable to believe that some small and humble rhinoviruses should be able to inhibit and partially stop the epidemiological development of a new pandemic influenza virus? In this context, the rhinoviruses may have another advantage, namely the large number of serotypes. It was discovered that more than 100 different rhinovirus types do not provide any mutual serological cross-protection. Most people experience several rhinovirus infections each year, whilst there may be several years in between before they acquire another respiratory virus like influenza.

The Virus Interference Hypothesis – an Old Idea

Interference between outbreaks of infection with RSV and influenza virus was first suggested by Glezen and co-worker in 1980 [8]. They observed that RSV outbreaks seemed interrupted by the onset of influenza virus infections. This was supported by Norwegian observations, which found that RSV and influenza virus outbreaks usually did not reach their epidemiological peaks during the same period [9]. Later studies have supported these findings [10,11]. It should, however, be mentioned that these observations are not unambiguous [12]. It may seem strange to talk about virus interference in the development of outbreaks with epidemic viruses. However, it is well known that if one mixes different viruses in cell cultures, this will result in virus interference, which will be exhibited as a reduced susceptibility of the cells for the last added virus. It was studies of these phenomena that led Isaacs and Lindemann to the discovery of interferon in 1957 [13]; a discovery that was later awarded with the Nobel Prize in medicine.

It is really unlikely that these phenomena will only be applicable in vitro and not in vivo [10]. All living organisms are subject to the evolution theories in which natural selection and everyone's struggle against all are key concepts.

Indeed, to word this in an apt and short way – it is unlikely that epidemic viruses should circulate freely and independently. If so, it would be contrary to essential elements in the evolution theories. Rather, the question should be: Is the actual virus in such a position that the mutual interference forces are exposed, and are our monitoring systems good enough to pick them up? Although virus interference remains a mere hypothesis, it provides a very plausible explanation why the Spanish flu and other influenza pandemics, in contrast to seasonal influenza, tend to occur in waves.

Viruses Are Like All of Us

A virus is considered to represent a border area between living and dead material. In many ways the interference hypothesis alters this picture – we see the outlines of features that are recognized in higher organisms, including *Homo sapiens*. Under normal conditions epidemic viruses "live" mostly in a harmonic coexistence with each other, but like many others things in life, they become "intriguing" and "jealous". This becomes evident when a newcomer tries to leave its intended place in the queue and gains a new place ahead.

Cytokines

How can the interference phenomena be explained? We have already mentioned interferon and a number of articles have suggested that the cytokine interferon is the most likely executor of this effect [2, 9, 10, 14]. Cytokines represent the human body's first line of fortification and are a part of the innate immune system.

Unlike the acquired immune system with its antibodies, the cytokines are not virus specific. That implies that during the short period after the host has suffered a rhinovirus or influenza virus infection he will be in an antiviral state, which renders him less susceptible to other virus infections.

References

[1] Norwegian Institute of Public Health (Folkehelseinstituttet). Available from http://www.fhi.no/influensa. (Accessed April 30, 2010).

[2] Linde A, Rotzén-Östlund M, Zweygberg-Wirgart B, Rubinova S, Brytting M. Does viral interference affect spread of influenza? *Euro. Surveill.* 2009;14:pii:19354.

[3] Ånestad G, Nordbø SA. Interference between outbreaks of respiratory viruses. *Euro. Surveill.* 2009;14:pii:19359.

[4] Ånestad G, Nordbø SA. Virus interference. Did rhinoviruses activity hamper the progress of the 2009 influenza A (H1N1) pandemic in Norway? *Med. Hypotheses* 2011;77:1132-4.

[5] Casalegno JS, Ottmann M, Bouscambert-Duchamp M, Valette M, Morfin F, Lina B. Impact of the 2009 influenza A(H1N1) pandemic wave on the pattern of hibernal respiratory virus epidemics, France, 2009. *Euro. Surveill.* 2010;15:pii:19485.

[6] Lower AC, Mubareka S, Steel J, Plese P. Influenza virus transmission is dependent on relative humidity and temperature. *PLoS Pathog.* 2007;3:1470-6.

[7] Greer RM, McErlean P, Arden, KE, Faux CE, Nitsche A, Lambert SB, Nissen MD, Sloots TP, Mackay IM. Do rhinoviruses reduce the probability of viral co-detection during acute respiratory tract infections? *J. Clin. Virol.* 2009;45:10-5.

[8] Glezen WP, Denny FW. Epidemiology of acute lower respiratory disease in children. *N. Engl. J. Med.* 1973;288:498-505.

[9] Ånestad G. Interference between outbreaks of respiratory syncytial virus and influenza virus infection. *Lancet* 1982;1:502.

[10] Ånestad G. Surveillance of respiratory viral infections by rapid immunofluorescence diagnosis, with emphasis on virus interference. *Epidemiol. Infect.* 1987;99:523-31.

[11] Ånestad G, Vainio K, Hungnes O. Interference between outbreaks of epidemic viruses. *Scand. J. Infect. Dis.* 2007;39:653-4.

[12] Ånestad G, Vainio K, Hungnes O. Interference between outbreaks of epidemic viruses: additional Norwegian observations. *Scand. J. Infect. Dis.* 2009;41:38.

[13] Isaacs A, Lindenmann J. Virus interference. I. The interferon. *Proc. R Soc. Lond B Biol. Sci.* 1957;147:258-67.

[14] Nishimura N, Nishio H, Lee MJ, Uemura K. The clinical features of respiratory syncytial virus: Lover respiratory tract infection after upper respiratory tract infection due to influenza virus. *Pediatr. Int.* 2005 47:412-6.

INDEX

C

D

E

F

G

H

I

J

K

L

M

N

O

P

R

S

T

U

V

W

Y